Vaginal Pessaries

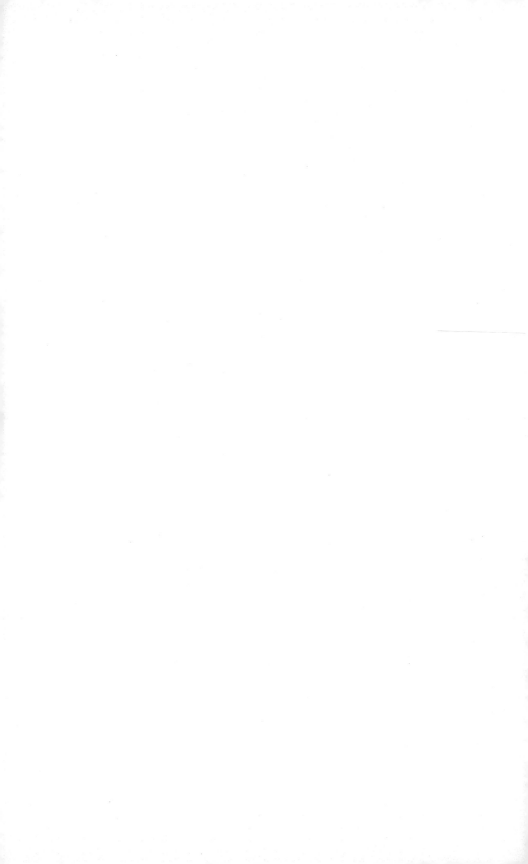

Vaginal Pessaries

Edited by

Teresa Tam, MD, FACOG, FACS

Gynecologist in private practice
All for Women Healthcare, SC
Chicago and Skokie, Illinois

Director of Minimally Invasive Gynecological Surgery
Amita Saint Francis Hospital
Evanston, Illinois

Assistant Professor of Obstetrics and Gynecology
Rush University Medical Center
Chicago, Illinois

Matthew F. Davies, MD, FACOG

Professor of Obstetrics and Gynecology
Penn State University

Chief of Female Pelvic Medicine and Reconstructive Surgery
Vice-Chair of Clinical Quality and Patient Safety and
Assistant Residency Program Director
Penn State Health
Milton S. Hershey Medical Center
Hershey, Pennsylvania

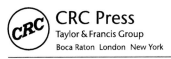
CRC Press
Taylor & Francis Group
Boca Raton London New York

CRC Press is an imprint of the
Taylor & Francis Group, an **informa** business

CRC Press
Taylor & Francis Group
6000 Broken Sound Parkway NW, Suite 300
Boca Raton, FL 33487-2742

© 2020 by Taylor & Francis Group, LLC
CRC Press is an imprint of Taylor & Francis Group, an Informa business

No claim to original U.S. Government works

Printed on acid-free paper

International Standard Book Number-13: 978-1-138-39440-7 (Paperback)
978-1-138-39441-4 (Hardback)

Library of Congress Cataloging-in-Publication Data

Names: Tam, Teresa, editor. | Davies, Matthew F., editor.
Title: Vaginal pessaries / edited by Teresa Tam, Matthew F. Davies.
Description: Boca Raton : CRC Press, [2020] | Includes bibliographical references and index. |
Summary: "With mesh surgery for prolapse sometimes proving problematic, there has been a resurgence of professional medical interest in more traditional methods for the management of prolapse and of stress urinary incontinence. This concise guide to the practical aspects of pessary use will be of interest to all gynecologists involved in clinical management of the patient with these problems"-- Provided by publisher.
Identifiers: LCCN 2019034050 (print) | LCCN 2019034051 (ebook) | ISBN 9781138394414 (hardback : alk. paper) | ISBN 9781138394407 (paperback : alk. paper) |
ISBN 9780429401183 (ebook)
Subjects: MESH: Pessaries
Classification: LCC RG137.3 (print) | LCC RG137.3 (ebook) | NLM WP 640 | DDC 618.1/85--dc23
LC record available at https://lccn.loc.gov/2019034050
LC ebook record available at https://lccn.loc.gov/2019034051

Visit the Taylor & Francis Web site at
http://www.taylorandfrancis.com

and the CRC Press Web site at
http://www.crcpress.com

I would like to thank Matthew Davies, MD, FACOG, for his mentorship and guidance, and Rick Hicaro for over 25 years of love and unwavering support.

—Teresa Tam

Contents

Preface

Vaginal pessaries have a long and colorful history, dating back to Egyptian times, the Middle Ages, and all the way to the age of modern medicine. However, despite advancements in the design and usage of pessaries over the ages, they had always taken a back seat to surgery in dealing with pelvic organ prolapse (POP) and stress urinary incontinence (SUI).

Enter the twenty-first century, when the focus on health care has moved toward preventative medicine and less invasive methodologies as alternatives to surgery. Patients will often seek treatments that are both less costly and less traumatic before considering the surgical option.

This is why the pessary has caught medical attention and public interest. With a wide variety of devices, both in design and fitment, the efficacy of pessary use has greatly improved over the pessaries of the past.

To date, very little has been written on the pessary. This book seeks to remedy that situation by providing a definitive resource for clinicians wishing to offer their patients this nonsurgical, minimally invasive treatment for their POP and SUI symptoms. It covers the many indications and the few contraindications for pessary usage, and routine maintenance (i.e., insertion/removal, sanitation, ongoing care, and patient follow-up management), all of which are key to successful pessary implementation. The full-color photos, tables, and illustrations show the different types of pessaries available to date, along with proper pessary fitting and care. Other indications of pessary use, including the cervical pessary, current clinical studies, and new inventions are also discussed.

The vaginal pessary offers a low-risk, cost-effective, nonsurgical treatment option for women of all ages with POP and SUI. It is an essential component of a clinician's armamentarium.

Vaginal Pessaries is the most concise, up-to-date, and much-needed compendium on the pessary and its application—highly appropriate for the state of health care in the twenty-first century. It serves as an invaluable reference for obstetrician–gynecologists, urogynecologists, urologists, primary care providers, and all other health care clinicians in the minimally invasive treatment of POP and SUI.

Teresa Tam
Matthew F. Davies

Acknowledgments

The editors would like to recognize Rick Hicaro who took the photos for the book cover. We also wish to thank Robert Peden of CRC Press/Taylor & Francis Group for his encouragement and invaluable suggestions throughout the process of creating this text.

Editors

Teresa Tam, MD, FACOG, FACS, is a board-certified obstetrician and gynecologist, fellowship trained in minimally invasive gynecological surgery (MIGS). She completed her MIGS fellowship and received advanced training in laparoscopic and robotic-assisted gynecological surgery at the Pennsylvania State University/Milton S. Hershey Medical Center. Along with her private practice, "All for Women Healthcare, SC," she is also the Director of Minimally Invasive Gynecological Surgery at Amita Saint Francis Hospital in Evanston and Assistant Professor of Obstetrics and Gynecology at Rush University Medical Center, Chicago, Illinois. Dr. Tam is a strong advocate for providing minimally invasive options such as the use of the vaginal pessary for pelvic organ prolapse and stress urinary incontinence. She believes the vaginal pessary is an important nonsurgical component of any clinician's gynecological armamentarium. Given her expertise, she has been invited annually since 2014 to be a clinical seminar speaker on the topic of vaginal pessary at the Annual Clinical Meeting of the American College of Obstetricians and Gynecologists (ACOG).

Matthew F. Davies, MD, FACOG, is a Professor of Obstetrics and Gynecology at the Pennsylvania State University as well as Chief of Female Pelvic Medicine and Reconstructive Surgery at Penn State Health–Milton S. Hershey Medical Center. His other roles are as Vice-Chair of Clinical Quality and Patient Safety and Assistant Residency Program Director. Formerly the Assistant Fellowship Director in Minimally Invasive Gynecologic Surgery, Dr. Davies' second fellow was Teresa Tam. Together they developed a video on pessary insertion techniques during her fellowship.

Contributors

Hayley Barnes, MD
Department of Obstetrics and
    Gynecology
Loyola University Medical Center
Maywood, Illinois

Sonia Bhandari Randhawa, MD
Department of Obstetrics and
    Gynecology
Reading Hospital
Reading, Pennsylvania

Sarah S. Boyd, MD
Department of Obstetrics and
    Gynecology
Division of Female Pelvic Medicine
    and Reconstructive Surgery
Penn State College of Medicine
Hershey, Pennsylvania

Kara Griffith, MD
Northwell Health
Hofstra University
Manhasset, New York

Marko J. Jachtorowycz, MD
AMITA Health Saint Francis Hospital
Evanston, Illinois
and
Metro Chicago Surgical Oncology, LLC
Wilmette, Illinois
and
University of Illinois College of
    Medicine
Chicago, Illinois

Kelly Jirschele, DO, FACOG, FACS
Illinois Urogynecology, Ltd.
Naperville, Illinois

Soo Kwon, MD
Northwell Health
Hofstra University
Lenox Hill Hospital
New York, New York

Jaime B. Long, MD
Department of Obstetrics and
    Gynecology
Division of Female Pelvic Medicine
    and Reconstructive Surgery
Penn State College of Medicine
Hershey, Pennsylvania

Michael D. Moen, MD, FACOG, FACS
Illinois Urogynecology, Ltd.
Park Ridge, Illinois

Thythy Pham, MD, MA
Department of Obstetrics and
    Gynecology
Loyola University Medical Center
Maywood, Illinois

Anne F. Wright, APN, WHNP-BC
Illinois Urogynecology, Ltd.
Park Ridge, Illinois

1

Historical Review

Jaime B. Long and Sonia Bhandari Randhawa

CONTENTS

Introduction

Pelvic organ prolapse (POP) and its different treatment options have been documented concerns for women through centuries of evolving civilizations. Pessaries, devices placed in the vagina to support the uterus or vaginal walls, have been a mainstay method of treatment for thousands of years. For most of this time, their use was guided by expert opinion and experience, but currently, there are better tools to improve their utilization. In addition to treating POP, pessaries have been used to treat urinary incontinence, uterine retroversion, and cervical insufficiency.

The term *pessary* is derived from the Greek word "pessos," which was an oval stone used in games. Homer described checkers-like games played with iron balls called "pessos" in *The Odyssey*.[1] It then evolved to describe oval stones that were placed in the uteri of camels for contraception in both Arabia and Turkey, and later was used to describe other intrauterine devices.[2]

Ancient Times

Over many centuries, various ancient civilizations including the Egyptians, Indians, Chinese, and Greeks have propagated their unique medications and remedies for the treatment of prolapse.[3] The change lies only in the materials and methods used to undergo this process. Both past and modern times are in agreement that the ideal conservative treatment of prolapse includes reducing the prolapsed organ with lubricating agents and placing objects into the vaginal canal to prevent recurrent prolapse.

The Kahun papyrus from ancient Egypt (2000 BC) portrayed the uterus as an independent animal, such as a tortoise, which was capable of movement within its host.[4] It recommended that women to stand over burning ingredients to force the prolapsed organs back into the vaginal canal.[4] Another early reference to the treatment of uterine and vaginal prolapse was found in the Ebers papyrus (1550 BC), which prescribed honey and petroleum applied to the finger of the patient and the uterus, which then pressed upon the prolapse and returned it to its position.[5] Fumes and aromatherapy were also used to fumigate the uterus, penetrating the uterine cavity and causing the uterus to return inside the body.[5]

During the time of Hippocrates, circa 400 BC, physicians employed many imaginative treatments including "succussion" therapy. This treatment entailed hanging the patient upside down from a ladder-like frame by her feet while being shaken up and down for 3–5 minutes. This procedure was an attempt to return the prolapsed organs back into the body with the assistance of gravitational force.[4] "Cupping" the buttocks and abdomen were also attempted in the hopes of returning the prolapsed organs to their proper position. Another approach was to use hot oil treatments to reduce the prolapse. If successful, pessaries consisting of wool soaked in an astringent were inserted in the vagina while the patient was prescribed bed rest. Another early pessary described by the Greek physician and author of the text *On Diseases of Women*, Polybus, involved the placement of half a pomegranate soaked in wine into the vagina.[3]

In AD 98, Soranus of Ephesus in his treatise *Gynaecology*, espoused the belief that placing herbs and various fumigations either on the patient's head or around the vagina would entice the organs to return to their areas of origin inside the body. Specifically, pleasant odors surrounded the patient's head to draw the uterus upward, while fetid odors were applied to the vagina to encourage the organ to ascend.[7]

Paulus Aegina (AD 600) utilized pessaries consisting of wool soaked in one of three different solutions: emollient, astringent, and anastomative.[5] Abbas in AD 932 wrote extensively on genital prolapse and treated it with manual reduction after placement of a wool pessary.[5] During this time, pieces of beef, as well as wooden plugs soaked in astringent vinegar, were utilized as pessaries. Trotula, the wife of Joannes Platearius (AD 1050), was the first female gynecologist. She prescribed a ball pessary made of strips of linen to fill the vagina and correct the prolapse.[5] Mechanical methods continued to be employed to keep pessaries in place, including leg binding and bed rest, with the feet elevated above the head.

These interventions for prolapse were not done in the absence of a basic anatomic understanding. In the second century AD, Aretaeus the Cappadocian described the uterine ligaments as the sails of a boat and explained that uterine prolapse was caused by relaxation of those very structures.[6]

Middle Ages (400–1400)

Until the sixteenth century, naturally occurring materials and objects continued to be utilized as pessaries; after that, devices were manufactured and created for the sole purpose of pessary use. The Middle Ages consequently saw limited innovation in the diagnosis and management of uterine prolapse.[6] By the end of the thirteenth century, Myrepus described the preparation of 45 different natural material pessaries with vastly varying elements. One interesting example, the Emmenagogue, consisted of a collection of ingredients including cumin, ginger, birthwort, and castor that were mixed with wax, honey, or suet.[5] Documents in the late 1300s showed that a uterus being extirpated does not necessarily equate to mortality. Marco Gattinara of Pavia first described this procedure.[6]

Sixteenth Century (1500–1599)

The first true vaginal hysterectomy was believed to have been performed by Berengario da Carpi in 1521, who utilized twine placed around the prolapsed uterus and gradually tightened over days until the organ was severed.[6] However, many physicians at the time continued to use pessaries, thus fostering emerging innovations. Bauhin, in the early 1500s, created a pessary that was a silver circle supported on a stalk with three branches, such that the ring was introduced into the superior part of the vagina and the cervix fixed into it.[7]

Ambrose Paré, a French surgeon of the European Renaissance, made oval-shaped pessaries from hammered brass or cork covered in wax. He also devised pear- and ring-shaped pessaries made of gold, silver, or brass that were held in place by a belt worn around the waist.[5] These belts were adjoined to apparatuses known as hysterophores. These consisted of a cup situated in the vagina to bear the uterus, which was then attached to four elastic tubes extending downward to unite in a leather plate to which the cup was fastened by a screw (Figure 1.1).[8] These apparatuses were often cumbersome to use and made movements such as standing and lying down very difficult.

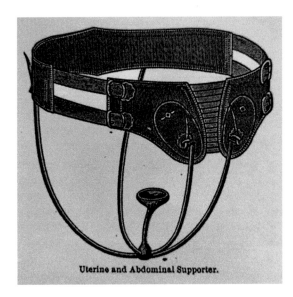

FIGURE 1.1 Pessary belt. (From Fritsch H. *The Diseases of Women. A Manual for Physicians and Students*. New York, NY: William Wood and Company, 1883. 214–223.)

Seventeenth Century (1600–1699)

Hendrik van Roonhuyse, a Dutch gynecologist who is credited with one of the earlier texts of operative obstetrics and gynecology, created a cork pessary with a hole in it to allow passage of vaginal discharge. He went on to describe one of the first complications and resolutions of pessary use by apparently removing a wax pessary that was obstructing a patient's lochia.[5] One of the more creative methods for managing prolapse described by R. de Castro in 1603 suggested "attacking it [the prolapse] with a piece of iron—red hot—as if to burn it, at which point fright will force the prolapsed part to recede into the vagina."[6]

Eighteenth Century (1700–1799)

In the 1700s, a more precise understanding arose regarding the problems related to prolapse and the surrounding organs.[6] In 1702, Saviard described the difference between prolapse and an inversion of a uterus.[6] The pessary of Saviard consisted of a steel spring, one end of which was fixed to a girdle and the other supported by a cushion and curved to reach just within the vagina and support the uterus.[7] During this period, Levret (a renowned obstetrician who was best known for his development of the Mauriceau-Levret maneuver for breech presentation delivery) first theorized that uterine prolapse resulted from the relaxation of ligaments of the peritoneum.[6,10]

The late seventeenth and eighteenth centuries also brought advanced clinical therapies and concoctions promoted to treat prolapse. Pessaries were made of varying shapes and new materials adapted to different POP diagnoses. Thomas Simson, a professor at the University of Edinburgh, created a metal spring that kept a cork ball pessary in place.[5] Jean Juville introduced soft rubber pessaries (shaped similar to contraceptive diaphragms) with a perforated gold tip that allowed for drainage. The pessary perforations addressed the issues of vaginal wall injuries that were common with metal pessaries.[9] Karl Mayer (founder of the first gynecologic clinic in Germany) created the Mayer pessary, a large soft rubber ring that retained the uterus in the pelvis by distending the upper part of the vagina.[9,11] August Breisky, an Austrian professor of obstetrics and gynecology, recommended large ovoid bodies of hard rubber. An innovative device by Maurice Gariel of France was an air-pessary consisting of a soft rubber bag that the patients would self-insert and fill with air at the time of use[9,12] (Figure 1.2).

The understanding of pessary-related complications such as pain with insertion and erosion into the vaginal canal continued to evolve. In 1710, European gynecologists Andreas Ottomar Goelicke and Johanne Georg Preunel invented a cone-shaped pessary covered in soft leather to provide

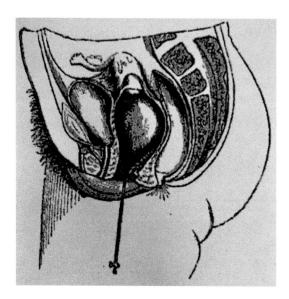

FIGURE 1.2 Air-pessary. (From Courty A. *Practical Treatise on the Diseases of the Uterus, Ovaries, and Fallopian Tubes.* London, England: J and A Churchill, 1882. 131–145.)

more comfort to the users. The pessary would be inserted while being pressed together and would then spring back into shape, once in the vagina, from its elasticity.[13] In 1750, obstetrician and gynecologist John Leake, the physician who replaced obstetric stools with delivery beds, introduced sponge pessaries, likewise to improve comfort and avoid complications from vaginal wall lacerations and erosions.[13,14] He documented a case report of a patient from whom he extracted a pessary that had eroded into the rectum, almost costing the patient her life.[13]

Nineteenth Century (1800–1899)

By the beginning of the nineteenth century, terminology and anatomic classification were introduced. The terminology is still commonly used today, including cystocele, rectocele, enterocele, and uterine prolapse/procidentia. Although surgical procedures and anesthesia were being refined, prolapse remained "exceedingly difficult to cure" surgically; therefore, a multitude of conservative methods for managing prolapse remained the mainstay of treatment. Friedrich Wilhelm Scanzoni, a German obstetrician (1856), recommended massage, as well as the local application of leeches, for excessive swelling. Others proposed cold water douches or "uterine gymnastics."[6]

E.E. Montgomery, a gynecologist from Jefferson Medical College, detailed the method of therapeutic massage as well as other conservative adjunctive prolapse care in his text *Practical Gynecology* (1901):

> Massage is practiced by placing the patient on a couch or bed, with the clothing loosened, introducing two fingers into the vagina, while the other hand is placed over the abdomen, the organ raised up against it, and with rotatory movements, the uterus is compressed between the two hands. The organ is grasped between the two hands, moved upward and downward, from side to side, and the bands of adhesion are stretched until sufficient irritation is induced to favor its reabsorption. This course of treatment should consist of seances of from five to ten minutes, two or three times a week. During the interval, the patient should use hot vaginal douches, rectal enemata, hot sitz baths, or the application of heat over the abdomen or pelvis in the form of a hot sand or peat. The treatment may be supplemented by the introduction of tampons medicated with glycerin, ichthyol, and glycerin, or ichthyol ointment. The tampon raises up the uterus and places it at a higher level, improves the circulation and promotes absorption. Massage has also an influence in stimulating the muscular activity of the ligaments in maintaining the organ in its proper place. Electricity may be applied in the form of galvanism or faradism. The former promotes the absorption of exudation; the latter develops the contractility of the muscular structure.

The pathophysiology of POP continued to be better understood. In his text *Diseases of Women* (1894), Henry Garrigues described the etiology as follows:

> The vaginal entrance being ruptured (from childbirth), the uterus does not find its usual support from below. It becomes retroverted and then retroflexed. Intra-abdominal pressure drives it like a wedge down through the vagina. The sacro-uterine ligaments become weakened and elongated, the pelvic connective tissue loses its tonus, and the weight of the subinvoluted vagina drags the uterus down. Finally, the uterus sinks by its own weight. Thus lack of support from above and below combines with weight, pressure and dragging to displace the uterus.

D. Berry Hart, a professor at the University of Edinburgh, in his 1883 *Manual of Gynecology*, hypothesized that prolapse originated from "lines of cleavage in the pelvic floor at which it separates or becomes dislocated under increased intra-abdominal pressure. Thus, strong pressure applied to the pelvic floor will cause it to bulge and displace all in front of the anterior rectal wall." He also suggested that a tear at the "sacral support segment" as well as a perineal tear are secondary factors in the etiology of prolapse.

By the mid-nineteenth century, the American Medical Association documented 123 different pessaries. There was also considerably more concern directed toward identifying a safer and more practical design. Hugh Lenox Hodge, in his book *Diseases Peculiar to Women*, extensively described the use of different pessaries. He suggested that the evils associated with pessaries arose from three sources: the material, the form, and the size of the instrument. Recommendations were made to use metal, glass, and porcelain pessaries instead of wood and cork, noting imminent and essential changes in pessary design. He also invented the lever pessary that would displace the cervix posteriorly, thus lifting the weight of the uterus off an incompetent cervix.[7]

In Howard Kelly's textbook (1896), he likewise emphasized the importance of material used, noting pessaries should always be made of hard rubber, not soft, as the latter becomes "foul and provokes vaginitis."[15] Additionally, he commented on the dimensions of the pessary, advising users to avoid tight rubber rings less than 6 mm in thickness, as these are more liable to cut through the vaginal walls.[15] He also cautioned against a "Horse Pessary," which he defined as a "large pessary which stretches the vaginal walls in every direction, liable to ulcerate living tissues."[15] An instrument known as a "Zwanck pessary" (Figure 1.3) was developed during this time with the purported advantage of improved retention through its expandable wings and stem. However, cases of injury and fistulae led to calls for its banishment by Kelly, Montgomery, and other contemporaries.[8] In addition, he advised

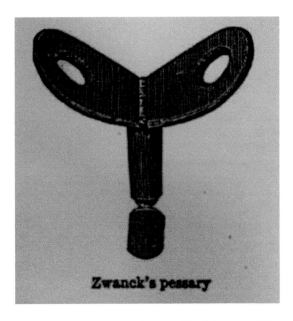

FIGURE 1.3   Zwanck pessary. (From Fritsch H. *The Diseases of Women. A Manual for Physicians and Students.* New York, NY: William Wood and Company, 1883. 214–223.)

pessary care with supervision including scheduled removal and cleaning, use of douches (borax, sodium bicarbonate, and menthol), and suppositories (boroglyceride, gelatin).

During this century, the ring (Figure 1.4), Munde, Schultze, Hodge, Smith, and Cutter pessaries also came into use.[5,16] The Hodge pessary had a broader anterior limb that prevented the pessary from turning and thereby precluding pressure on the urethra.[5] The Smith pessary was created with a narrower anterior limb for application in a patient with a narrow pubic arch (Figure 1.5).

The Cutter pessary had a crescentic bar, a loop, or a cup mounted on a stem having a perineal curve (Figure 1.6). From this apparatus stemmed a piece of rubber tubing which was connected with a strap that buckled onto a waist belt.[17] The limitation of this pessary was the difficulty adjusting the top of the pessary as it hit against the uterus.

Furthermore, the tubing would easily get dirty. These problems limited its use.[17] The cup and stem pessary also had multiple variations with similar straps at the base and an expanded head that formed a platform on which the uterus rested.[17] Patients were instructed to remove these pessaries every night and to replace the straps as necessary because the material was often cheap and easily soiled (Figure 1.7).[17]

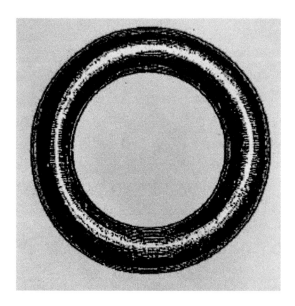

FIGURE 1.4 Ring pessary. (From Montgomery EE. *Practical Gynecology.* Philadelphia, PA: Blakiston's Son and Co., 1901. 429–437.)

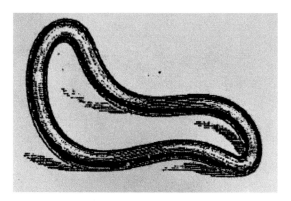

FIGURE 1.5 Smith-Hodge pessary. (From Montgomery EE. *Practical Gynecology.* Philadelphia, PA: Blakiston's Son and Co., 1901. 429–437.)

Modern Times (1900–Now)

There has been significant refinement and improvement in the pessaries of today. Perhaps the most significant advancement of pessaries in the twentieth century was replacing the rubber used in pessaries with polystyrene (circa 1950). Modern pessaries of today are often made of silicone and rarely of

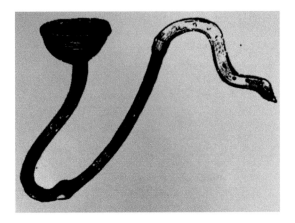

FIGURE 1.6   Cutter pessary. (From Herman GE. *JAMA*. 1914;LXII[2]:152.)

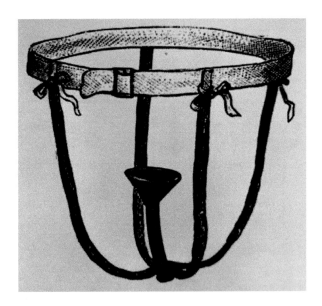

FIGURE 1.7   Cup and stem pessary. (From Herman GE. *JAMA*. 1914;LXII[2]:152.)

latex or acrylic. Silicone is noted to be advantageous because it is flexible yet sturdy, hypoallergenic, and durable. It has a relatively long half-life, is resistant to repetitive cleaning, and is relatively nonabsorbent to secretions and odors that surround it on a daily basis.[5]

Numerous shapes and sizes of pessaries currently exist to fit the individual needs of women around the world, each with its advantages and disadvantages.

The ring pessary, while easy to insert and allows for coitus, requires patient compliance and is better suited for women with less severe uterovaginal prolapse.[5] The Gellhorn pessary enables large prolapses to be kept in place; however, it is rigid and difficult to insert. The donut pessary is popular due to its excellent supportive properties but again is more difficult to insert and remove. The cube pessary, useful in women who lack vaginal tonicity, is challenging to manage as it requires nightly removal to drain secretions and relieve tissue ischemia from suction properties.[5]

The donut pessary originated from the Schatz pessary, described in 1905, which was created by Professor Schatz while working at Rostock University in Mecklenburg, Germany.[18] It was developed as a saucer-shaped pessary made of hard rubber and perforated in the center to allow for secretions to pass through.[7] From the time of its inception, it was created in multiple sizes and was developed to be retained in cases of prolapse or procidentia, even with torn perineum and loose vaginal walls.[18]

The Gellhorn pessary was created by George Gellhorn, a gynecologist of German descent, who began practicing at St. Louis University and Washington University in 1899.[19] The Gehrung pessary was introduced by another St. Louis obstetrician and gynecologist, Eugene Gehrung, in 1880.[20] The Gehrung support pessary was developed as an anteversion pessary to straighten and lift the anteflexed uterus as a "double horseshoe" (Figure 1.8).[20] The lower arch rests on the floor of the pelvis, and the uterus reclines on the superior curve. Today, the Gehrung pessary is available in multiple sizes and continues to be positioned with the convexity of the curved bars toward the anterior vaginal wall. It is used to provide support for rectocele, cystocele, and procidentia.[3]

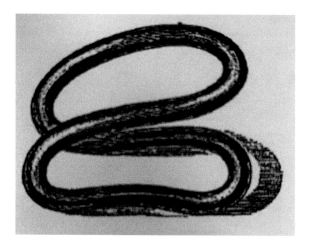

FIGURE 1.8 Gehrung pessary. (From Montgomery EE. *Practical Gynecology.* Philadelphia, PA: Blakiston's Son and Co., 1901. 429–437.)

Although reliance on the mechanical methods of prolapse reduction has decreased with the advent of modern surgical techniques, vaginal pessaries remain an immensely useful and safe treatment option for POP.[3] Up to 75% of specialist clinicians offer pessaries as their first-line treatment because of their high effectiveness without surgical risks.[21] A randomized controlled trial of pessary use in women with symptomatic POP (pelvic floor exercise versus pessary + pelvic floor exercise) noted that pessaries improve pelvic floor symptoms as well as correct hydronephrosis in women with POP.[21] This group asserted that pessaries are effective in women with various stages of prolapse and should not only be offered to poor surgical candidates.

Conclusion

POP has been a medical concern affecting the lives of countless women through evolving civilizations and varying cultures. Early treatment attempts and rituals were improved as physicians developed a better understanding of human anatomy and the pathophysiology of POP. The use of vaginal pessaries has evolved as the mainstay of conservative treatment for POP. Knowledge of the disease process improved over time to include various forms, degrees, and organs involved. New eras brought forward innovative materials and methods to reach modern-day pessaries, which are primarily made of silicone in varying shapes and sizes for increased hygiene and ease of use. Advancements in form, technique, and material have made the pessaries of today a viable and safe alternative to surgery for POP and urinary incontinence, significantly improving the quality of life for many women.[2] They are used not only for women who are poor surgical candidates but also for women who wish to have a nonsurgical treatment.

REFERENCES

1. Tait L. *Diseases of Women*. New York, NY: William Wood and Company, 1879. 86–87.
2. Chen CCG, Long J. Nonsurgical management of pelvic organ prolapse. In: Jones HW, Rock JA, eds, *Te Linde's Operative Gynecology*. 11th edition. Philadelphia. PA: Wolters Kluwer, 2015. 904–911.
3. Oliver R. The history and usage of the vaginal pessary: A review. *EJOG*. 2010;155(2):125–130.
4. Tizzano A. The history and evolution of sutures in pelvic surgery. *J R Soc Med*. 2011 Mar;104(3):107–112.
5. Shah SM, Sultan AH, Thakar R. The history and evolution of pessaries for pelvic organ prolapse. *Int Urogynecol J*. 2006;17:170–175.

6. Emge LA, Durfee RB. Pelvic organ prolapse: Four thousand years of treatment. *Clin Obstet Gynecol.* 1966 Dec;9(4):997–1032.

7. Churchill F. *Outlines of the Principle Diseases for Females.* Dublin, Ireland: William Warren, 1835. 79–81.

8. Fritsch H. *The Diseases of Women. A Manual for Physicians and Students.* New York, NY: William Wood and Company, 1883. 214–223.

9. Garrigues HJ. *A Text-Book of the Diseases of Women.* Philadelphia, PA: W.B. Saunders, 1894. 440–447.

10. Karamanou M. André Levret (1703–1780): The eminent obstetrician of the 18th century and his innovative approach to the treatment of uterine polyps. *JBUON.* 2017;22(2):562–565.

11. Waite L. *The Medical Standard, Volume 29.* Chicago, IL: G.P. Engelhard and Co., 1906. 45–57.

12. Courty A. *Practical Treatise on the Diseases of the Uterus, Ovaries, and Fallopian Tubes.* London, England: J and A Churchill, 1882. 131–145.

13. Ricci JV. *The Development of Gynæcological Surgery and Instruments.* Toronto, Canada: The Blakiston Company, 1949. 148–185.

14. Jacob A. *A Comprehensive Textbook of Midwifery and Gynecological Nursing.* 3rd edition. New Delhi, India: Jaypee Brothers Medical Publishers, 2012. 718–765.

15. Kelly HA. *Medical Gynecology.* New York, NY: D. Appleton and Company, 1908. 299–316.

16. Montgomery EE. *Practical Gynecology.* Philadelphia, PA: Blakiston's Son and Co, 1901. 429–437.

17. Herman, GE. Diseases of women. A clinical guide to their diagnosis and treatment. *JAMA.* 1914;LXII(2):152.

18. Foster, F. *New York Medical Journal*, Volume 82. New York, NY: A. R. Elliot Publishing Company, 1905. 71–79.

19. Sicherman, B, Green, CH. *Notable American Women the Modern Period: A Biographical Dictionary.* Cambridge, MA: The Belkap Press of Harward University Press, 1980. 48–92.

20. Unde, PF. *Minor Surgical Gynecology, A Treatise of Uterine Diagnosis and the Lesser Technicalities of Gynecological Practice*, Volume 2. New York, NY: William Wood and Company, 1885. 387–389.

21. Cheung RY. Vaginal pessary in women with symptomatic pelvic organ prolapse. *Obstet Gynecol.* 2016 Jul;128(1):73–80.

2

Pessaries for Pelvic Organ Prolapse

Michael D. Moen and Anne F. Wright

CONTENTS

Pelvic organ prolapse (POP), defined as descent of the uterus and/or walls of the vagina, is a common condition in adult women and can cause multiple symptoms including a sensation of vaginal pressure or bulge, heaviness or dragging sensation in the pelvis, difficulty urinating and evacuating stool, and dyspareunia. Risk factors for POP include prior vaginal delivery and its associated pelvic floor trauma, obesity, chronic straining due to constipation or heavy lifting due to work-related activities, chronic coughing due to diseases such as asthma or chronic obstructive pulmonary disease (COPD), and connective tissue disorders. Patients with POP often report that, due to their symptoms, they are no longer able to engage in the activities they enjoy most. They are hesitant to travel, exercise, go on extended walks, or even continue to work at a long-held job. Symptoms related to POP can affect quality of life (QOL), and women with POP have a negative body image compared to women without POP.[1]

Treatment options for POP include conservative management and surgical correction. Some elements to consider when deciding on appropriate treatment are the degree of prolapse, the severity of the symptoms, and the health status of the patient. Simple observation of prolapse may be an option for women with mild prolapse and minimal symptoms. Similarly, pelvic floor muscle strengthening with Kegel exercises can be attempted along with lifestyle modification such as avoiding constipation, weight loss (if indicated), avoidance of heavy lifting and high-impact exercise, and smoking cessation.[2]

For more advanced or bothersome prolapse affecting QOL, many patients will seek surgical correction as a treatment option. A pessary is an excellent option for women with bothersome POP who are awaiting surgery, are not motivated to undergo surgery, or are not surgical candidates based on health status. For these women, placement of a vaginal pessary is the standard nonsurgical option to alleviate symptoms and offers a low-risk and relatively inexpensive treatment option. Contraindications to pessary placement include any type of active vaginal infection, vaginal ulceration or lesion, or severe vaginal atrophy.

Historically, POP has been addressed for hundreds if not thousands of years with objects inserted into the vagina including cloth, wood, wax, metal, ivory, spheres made of bone or gold, as well as twine shaped into a ball and pomegranates soaked in vinegar. References to the use of such objects appear in early Egyptian hieroglyphics and in books about midwifery in the seventeenth century.[3] Although pessaries have historically been made from many different materials, they are now made from silicone, acrylic, latex, or rubber. The most common types currently used are silicone pessaries, which offer the most benefit because they are flexible, long lasting, nonabsorbent of odors, nonallergenic, and washable.[4] Several clinical trials have been reported in which pessaries were found to relieve bothersome symptoms of prolapse.[5–8]

Pessaries for POP generally can be placed into two categories. The first are support pessaries that rely on support from the patient's own pelvic floor muscles. The most common support pessaries used are the ring pessary, ring with support pessary, and the Shaatz pessary (Figure 2.1). Additional support pessaries include the Hodge pessary and the Gehrung pessary. The second category of pessaries are space-occupying pessaries. These include the Gellhorn and Cube pessaries (Figure 2.2), which are the most common space-occupying pessaries used currently. These pessaries are concave in shape and form a suction against the vaginal walls, making them more likely to stay in place. Additional space-occupying pessaries include the donut pessary and the inflatable pessary. Traditionally, space-occupying pessaries have been

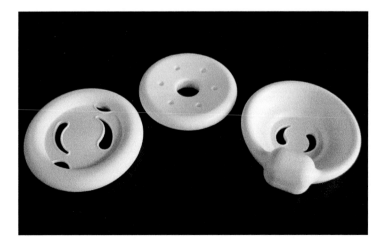

FIGURE 2.1   Ring with support, Shaatz, and incontinence dish pessaries.

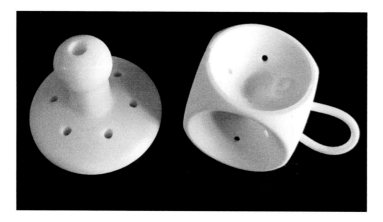

FIGURE 2.2 Gellhorn and cube pessaries.

recognized as the choice for more advanced prolapse and are known to increase the risk of vaginal epithelial injury. These pessaries may preclude intercourse while in place. They are also more difficult for both the patient and the provider to remove and reinsert.

In addition to support and space-occupying pessaries, there are also pessaries designed to treat stress incontinence. These include the incontinence ring, the incontinence dish, and the incontinence dish with support. Because these pessaries have a knob or ridge located anteriorly, they can be used in patients who have anterior compartment prolapse (cystocele).

Studies indicate that pessaries are a common treatment modality and are used in daily practice by more than 86% of nurse providers and gynecologists and 98% of urogynecologists.[9–11] Despite the widespread use of pessaries in daily clinical practice, most providers receive little, if any, formal training in the art of pessary fitting.

Because there is a lack of consistent predictors for successful pessary fittings, it is assumed by many providers that all women seeking treatment for POP are potential candidates for a pessary trial. As mentioned previously, patient lifestyle often guides the provider's selection of pessary type. For example, patients interested in self-care of the device may be better suited with a pessary that is easy to remove and reinsert. Other patients with physical limitations such as arthritis, obesity, or difficulty with mobility may be better suited with a pessary that is more difficult to remove but provides less chance of spontaneous expulsion.

Specific parameters for pessary selection are difficult to define, and selection of pessary type and size is usually based on the physical exam. Therefore, the provider's clinical judgment, manufacturer guidelines, and patient preference are all relied upon. During pelvic exam, the vaginal depth and caliber are assessed to make an estimate of the appropriate-size pessary needed.

Most providers use the ring with support pessary as their first option. For ring pessary placement, the pessary is folded in half, and lubricant is applied to the leading portion of the pessary that will be inserted. It is helpful to grasp the pessary with the thumb and forefinger for insertion. The proper positioning for support pessaries is in the upper portion of the vagina, above the level of the pelvic floor muscles. For removal, the thumb and forefinger are used to grasp the edge of the pessary, and it is sometimes helpful to twist the pessary as it is being removed. This will help to fold the pessary as it is pulled through the vaginal canal. Another maneuver that can help patients with pessary removal is to tie a loop of dental floss to the pessary, which can then be grasped to help pull the pessary into the lower vaginal canal and allow the pessary to be grasped more easily. The goal of pessary fitting is to find the largest size that is comfortable. A pessary that is too small has a higher likelihood of being expelled or shifting while in place. This can cause discomfort and increases the risk of trauma to the vaginal epithelium, which can cause genital abrasions and ulcerations.

The majority of patients can be managed with a ring with support pessary. When this type is not successful, a Gellhorn-type pessary is used. The Gellhorn is more difficult to insert and remove but typically stays in place sufficiently to relieve POP in those patients who are not successful with ring pessaries. For insertion, the round, upper portion of the Gellhorn is folded toward the stem and inserted vertically in the same fashion used to insert a ring-type pessary. For removal, it is very helpful to grasp the knob end of the Gellhorn with a single-toothed tenaculum or ring forceps to assist with the necessary force needed to pull the pessary through the vagina. While gently providing traction on the instrument with one hand, the forefinger of the other hand can be inserted and used to break the suction that typically occurs between the vaginal wall and the disc portion of the Gellhorn pessary.

As with support pessaries, a properly positioned Gellhorn pessary should have the disc portion of the pessary in the upper vagina with the stem extending into the lower vaginal canal. Cube pessaries are also designed to be positioned in the upper vagina and have the advantage of an attached string or loop to help with removal, allowing some patients to self-manage their pessary. We encourage removal of cube pessaries one to two times each week to help minimize vaginal discharge and ulceration.

Pessary fitting is essentially a trial-and-error process, and providers should be aware that it may be necessary to try several different types and sizes of pessaries to achieve a successful fitting. The ultimate goal is simply to relieve the most bothersome symptoms, provide comfort to the patient, ensure the pessary remains in place during toileting, does not cause injury to vaginal epithelium, and does not cause obstruction to voiding or defecation. An interesting concept that may result in improved success for future pessary fitting is the use of three-dimensional printing technology to create custom pessaries for individual patients.[12]

Frequently Asked Questions

Once fitted with a pessary, patients often ask similar questions regarding pessary care and use. Patients often want to know what the pessary will feel like while in place, whether or not they are able to have intercourse without removing the device, or what they should do if the pessary falls out. Others may ask what they should do if the pessary becomes uncomfortable or if they can remove the pessary on their own. Patient education content includes providing the answers to these frequently asked questions (FAQs) at the time of the first visit or at a scheduled follow-up visit during which time is set aside specifically to teach patients self-management of the device. During these visits, patients are taught that pessaries can be worn all day or only at times when increased activity is anticipated, such as exercising or prolonged standing. Patients are advised that the pessary should typically not be felt while in place if optimally fitted. If the device is painful or falls out easily, patients should make an appointment to be fitted with a new pessary size or shape.

Care of the pessary is a vital component to pessary care teaching (Figure 2.3). Patients need to know that cleaning the pessary requires only a mild soap and water. There is no need to sterilize the device by boiling it or using any type of chemicals like bleach. If a patient is comfortable with self-care (removal and reinsertion), the patient is encouraged to remove the device once or twice a month, leave it out overnight, and reinsert in the morning. If a patient prefers to return to the office to have a health care provider perform removal, cleaning, and reinsertion, this should be scheduled on a regular basis, roughly every 3 months but can be individualized based on the patient's specific situation and needs. At this visit, the provider will perform a vaginal exam checking for vaginal discharge, erosions, or ulcerations, and evaluating for vaginal atrophy. If a patient is found to have any type of vaginal ulceration, a recommendation will be made that the pessary be left out for approximately 2 weeks to allow the vagina to heal. The patient may also be advised to use vaginal estrogen cream as part of their routine to improve the vaginal mucosa and prevent breakdown from pessary placement. If a foul-smelling discharge is noted, it may represent bacterial vaginosis, and an antibiotic such as metronidazole can be prescribed (Table 2.1).

Patients need to know when a call to their health care provider is warranted. These scenarios would include any signs of vaginal bleeding; pain with walking, sitting, or positional changes; foul-smelling or discolored discharge; an ill-fitting pessary that keeps falling out or slipping down; or one that no longer provides adequate support as evidenced by the prolapse going beyond the pessary.

Occasionally, the placement of a pessary may result in the new finding of stress urinary incontinence that was formerly masked by an obstructed urethra.

What is a pessary?

A pessary is a common and effective medical device, which has been used for centuries, to relieve symptoms of pelvic organ prolapse. Pessaries come in a variety of shapes and sizes and can be used for long-term, conservative management of prolapse.

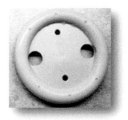

Caring for the Pessary

Self-Care	Clinic-Based Care
▪ Wash hands before caring for pessary ▪ Remove the pessary once per week ▪ Wash with soapy water ▪ Rinse well ▪ Leave out overnight and replace in the morning	▪ Follow-up in clinic every 3 months ▪ Monitoring of symptoms ▪ Exam for any possible skin breakdown ▪ Cleaning of pessary ▪ Reinsertion

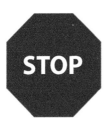

Warning Signs for Follow-Up

- Pain
- Bleeding
- Malodorous discharge
- Difficulty urinating or defecating
- Device falling out
- Vaginal atrophy (breakdown of the skin tissue)

FIGURE 2.3 Pessary care reference guide.

Elevation of the vaginal bulge can essentially "un-kink" the urethra and result in the patient having to deal with a new symptom of stress urinary incontinence. Often this problem, termed *occult stress incontinence*, is revealed at the time of new pessary placement. In other cases, it may become more apparent a day after pessary placement. This new finding can be distressing to patients and is often cited as a cause for discontinuation of pessary use. There are pessaries, which are specifically indicated for patients with occult stress incontinence. These include the incontinence ring and the incontinence dish pessaries. If these pessaries are successful, QOL-reducing symptoms of incontinence and prolapse are both addressed, and patients often choose to continue pessary use.

TABLE 2.1

Pessary Care Troubleshooting

Problem or Symptom	Possible Cause(s)	Remedies
Pessary will not stay in place: falls out, will not maintain correct orientation	Pessary too small	Try a larger size pessary
	Pessary design incompatible with anatomy	Try a different type of pessary
Pain or discomfort	Ill-fitting pessary (too small or too large)	Remeasure and refit pessary
	Mismatched pessary (incompatible design)	Try different type of pessary
Discharge or odor	Possible bacterial vaginosis	Treat with antibiotic (e.g., metronidazole cream)
		Consider use of vaginal estrogen (cream, tablet, ring)
Bleeding	Granulation tissue	Treat granulation tissue (e.g., silver nitrate)
	Ulcerations	Discontinue use until ulcerations heal
		Consider use of vaginal estrogen (cream, tablet, ring)
		Pelvic ultrasound for patients with a uterus to rule out a uterine source for bleeding
Anterior compartment prolapses (pessary in place)	Too small	Try a larger pessary
	Mismatched pessary (incompatible design)	Try different type of pessary
Stress incontinence (pessary is in place)	Pessary design	Try incontinence pessary (incontinence dish, ring with knob)
Unable to remove ring pessary	Difficulty reaching pessary	Dental floss can be tied around the rim of the pessary to create a loop assisting pessary removal

Conclusion

POP is a common condition that can significantly impact a woman's quality of life. Pessaries have been successfully used for years to treat the symptoms of POP. These devices have evolved into a variety of shapes and sizes that can be fitted to address various needs and lifestyles. When fitted successfully with a pessary, women report high satisfaction rates and improved perceptions of body image. Therefore, successful pessary placement can make a marked impact on reducing symptoms and improving QOL. The health care resources needed to address and treat POP are expected to rise due to the growing elderly population. Health care providers need to be educated on the various types, uses, and complications associated with pessary usage.

REFERENCES

1. Jelovsek JE, Barber MD. Women seeking treatment for advanced pelvic organ prolapse have decreased body image and quality of life. *Am J Obstet Gynecol.* 2006;194:1455–1461.
2. Nutt BS, Chaney S, Hill C. Diagnosis and management of pelvic organ prolapse the basics. *Women's Healthcare.* 2016;4:38–42.
3. Shah SM, Sultan AH, Thaker R. The history and evolution of pessaries for pelvic organ prolapse. *Int Urogynecol J.* 2006;17:170–175.
4. Atnip S, O'Dell K. Vaginal support pessaries: Indications for use and fitting strategies. *Urol Nurs.* 2012;32:114–124.
5. Clemons JL, Aguilar VC, Tillinghast TA, Jackson ND, Myers DL. Patient satisfaction and changes in prolapse and urinary symptoms in women who were fitted successfully with a pessary for pelvic organ prolapse. *Am J Obstet Gynecol.* 2004;90:1025–1029.
6. Fernando RJ, Thakar R, Sultan AH, Shah SM, Jones PW. Effect of vaginal pessaries on symptoms associated with pelvic organ prolapse. *Obstet Gynecol.* 2006;108:93–99.
7. Cheung RYK, Lee JHS, Lee LL, Chung TKH, Chan SSC. Vaginal pessary in women with symptomatic pelvic organ prolapse: A randomized controlled trial. *Obstet Gynecol.* 2016;128:73–80.
8. Yimphong T, Temtanakitpaison T, Buppasri P, Chongsomchai C, Kanchaiyaphum S. Discontinuation rate and adverse events after 1 year of vaginal pessary use in women with pelvic organ prolapse. *Int Urogynecol J.* 2018;29:1123–1128.
9. O'Dell K, Atnip S, Hooper G, Leung K. Pessary practices of nurse-providers in the United States. *Female Pelvic Med Reconstr Surg.* 2016;22:261–266.
10. Pott-Grinstein E, Newcomer JR. Gynecologists' patterns of prescribing pessaries. *J Repro Med.* 2001;46:205–208.
11. Cundiff GW, Weidner AC, Visco AG, Bump RC, Addison WA. A survey of pessary use by members of the American Urogynecologic Society. *Obstet Gynecol.* 2000;95:931–935.
12. Barsky M, Kelley R, Bhora FY, Hardart A. Customized pessary fabrication using three-dimensional printing technology. *Obstet Gynecol.* 2018;131:493–497.

3

Incontinence Pessaries

Sarah S. Boyd

CONTENTS

Background

Urinary incontinence is a common quality-of-life condition affecting women of all ages globally.[1] Stress urinary incontinence (SUI) is involuntary leakage of urine in the setting of increased abdominal pressure, such as laughing, coughing, sneezing, or exercise. Symptoms of SUI affect anywhere from 4% to 80% of women,[2–4] with 4%–11% undergoing surgery.[4,5] Incontinence pessaries are a safe and effective option in women desiring nonsurgical management or in whom medical comorbidities preclude surgery. In recent years, their use has also extended into pregnancy. The existence of nonsurgical options for the management of SUI is often a relief for these patients and should be a topic of discussion when counseling women on their various treatment options.

Types of Incontinence Pessaries

Pessaries used for the treatment of incontinence are most commonly support pessaries. They are thought to restore continence by stabilizing the proximal urethra and urethrovesical junction. Incontinence pessaries act as a backstop for the urethra during times of increased abdominal pressure.

TABLE 3.1

Types of Incontinence Pessaries with Indications

Type of Incontinence Pessary	Indication
Incontinence ring	For stress urinary incontinence (SUI) only
Incontinence dish	For SUI with mild prolapse
Incontinence dish with support	For SUI with mild prolapse and a mild cystocele
Ring with knob	Mild prolapse complicated by SUI
Ring with support and knob	Mild prolapse complicated by a mild cystocele and SUI
Hodge	For SUI + narrow vaginal introitus
Hodge with support	For SUI and mild cystocele + narrow vaginal introitus
Hodge with knob	For SUI + narrow vaginal introitus
Hodge with support and knob	For SUI complicated by mild cystocele + narrow vaginal introitus
Smith	For SUI + well-defined pubic notch
Gehrung with knob	For cystocele +/− mild rectocele complicated by SUI

According to the most recent Cooper Surgical, Inc. (Trumball, Connecticut) pessary guide, there are approximately 11 different incontinence pessaries available, ranging in size from 1¾ to 5 inches, depending on the pessary (Table 3.1).[6] Each style of incontinence pessary is designed to serve specific functions and patient needs. This allows the treatment of multiple pelvic floor disorders concomitantly in women with variations in pelvic anatomy. For example, incontinence dishes and rings are most commonly used in the straightforward patient with SUI only (Figure 3.1). If the patient also has pelvic organ prolapse quantification (POPQ) stage 1 anterior vaginal wall prolapse, an incontinence dish with support may be more appropriate (Figure 3.2).

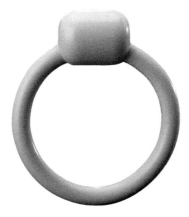

FIGURE 3.1   Incontinence ring pessary. (Courtesy of CooperSurgical, Inc.)

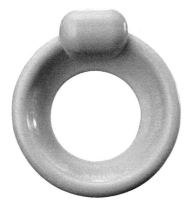

FIGURE 3.2   Incontinence dish pessary. (Courtesy of CooperSurgical, Inc.)

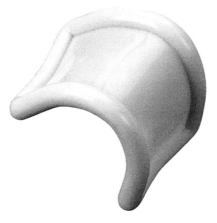

FIGURE 3.3   Gehrung pessary. (Courtesy of CooperSurgical, Inc.)

The patient with a narrow vaginal introitus may be most comfortable with a Hodge pessary with or without support or a knob, while the presence of a POPQ stage 1 posterior wall prolapse may prove the Gehrung pessary with knob to be the most effective (Figure 3.3).

Pessary Fitting and Management

The patient should be examined in a dorsal lithotomy position. The patient is instructed to refrain from voiding before the fitting to allow a pre- and post-fitting supine cough stress test. This will enable the clinician to assess continence with the pessary in place. There is no consensus on the optimal technique to estimate the initial pessary size, and several sizes and types may need to be attempted.[5,7] We gauge the initial sizing using the POPQ point GH, or genital hiatus. After determining the approximate size, the appropriate incontinence pessary is chosen based on the patient's needs, activity level, and pelvic anatomy as described previously. Incontinence rings and dishes with and without support, depending on the presence of concomitant pelvic organ prolapse, are commonly used as they are easiest to fold, insert, and remove. These characteristics also allow feasibility in self-management should the patient desire.

With dry gloves to allow better stabilization of the pessary, the pessary should be folded. The clinician can use water-soluble lubricants at the leading edge of the pessary as needed. Except for the Hodge, Hodge with support, and Smith incontinence pessary, the remaining incontinence pessaries shown in Table 3.1 incorporate a protrusion called a "knob" on one edge. The knob is oriented most distal in the vagina to lay under the urethra and directly behind the symphysis pubis. The edge directly opposite the knob side of the pessary is the leading edge—this opposing side is oriented most proximal in the vagina, introduced first when placing a pessary (Figure 3.4). It is at this proximal, leading edge to which lubrication is applied at the time of insertion. The pessary is inserted past the introitus and should be guided posteriorly to avoid the urethra and rest behind the symphysis pubis (Figure 3.5). An appropriately sized pessary should allow the clinician to easily sweep his or her index finger between the pessary and the vaginal wall. The pessary should feel comfortable for the patient; it should not shift when the patient is active. The patient should be instructed to stand, ambulate, Valsalva, and cough to ensure the pessary is retained (see Chapter 4). A supine cough stress test is repeated after placement to ensure adequate urethral support and continence. Last, the clinician should ensure the patient could void with the pessary in place before discharge home.

Self-management of the pessary should be discussed and encouraged based on patient preference and ability. Patients are instructed to remove and insert

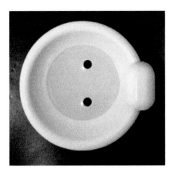

FIGURE 3.4   Orientation of incontinence pessary for fitting. Incontinence dish with support and knob, 80 mm size with knob on right and leading edge on left.

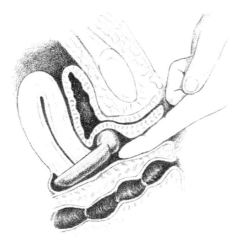

FIGURE 3.5   Proper insertion of an incontinence pessary. (Courtesy of CooperSurgical, Inc.)

the pessary either standing or supine based on their dexterity and comfort level. We recommend cleaning the pessary with soap and water each time it is removed and using water-soluble lubricants as needed.

Follow-Up Recommendations

After the initial fitting, we recommend a follow-up appointment within 2–4 weeks for assessment of comfort and continuation. After that, the patient is seen at 3- to 6-month intervals if she prefers the clinician to remove and clean the pessary or 6- to 12-month intervals if self-managing. Follow-up visits should include an assessment of pain, comfort, and continence. The clinician should inquire about the presence of vaginal bleeding and discharge. The examination should include evaluation of the vaginal wall for epithelial abnormalities including granulation tissue, pressure sores, ulcerations, and atrophy. Pessary size and type should also be evaluated with changes made as needed based on patient symptoms and examination.

Efficacy of Pessaries for Stress Urinary Incontinence

Incontinence pessaries are feasible, safe, and effective for the treatment of SUI in women desiring nonsurgical management. Small studies on short-term outcomes with incontinence pessaries show an improvement in urinary symptoms, body image perception, and sexual function.[5,7-13] However, there is a paucity of data on long-term outcomes or high-quality prospective trials comparing incontinence pessaries with other nonsurgical therapies.

One large, prospective trial by the Pelvic Floor Disorders Network published in 2010 randomized 446 women with SUI to pessary, behavioral therapy, or combined treatment and measured the patients' impression of improvement and SUI using the Pelvic Floor Distress Inventory (PFDI).[14] Improvement at 3 months was similar between pessary and behavioral groups with 40% and 49% reporting "much better" or "very much better," while more women in the behavioral group reported no incontinence symptoms and treatment satisfaction compared to the pessary group.[14] Patient satisfaction remained more than 50% for all groups at 12 months.[14] A subsequent secondary analysis of this trial showed successful treatment of SUI was associated with improvement in sexual function by a validated questionnaire, improvement in incontinence with sexual activity, and greater reduction in restriction in sexual activity due to fear of incontinence.[8] While incontinence pessaries may not be superior to other nonsurgical therapies, they are proven to be successful in the management of SUI and associated with high patient satisfaction. This further emphasizes the importance of counseling patients on their effectiveness if considering a nonsurgical modality for SUI treatment.

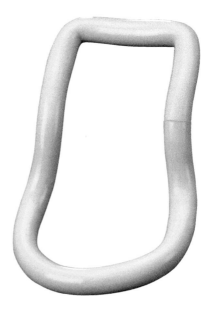

Hodge lever pessary. (Courtesy of CooperSurgical, Inc.)

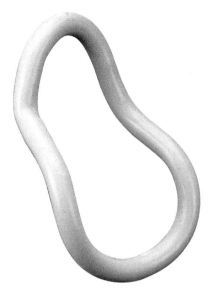

Smith lever pessary. (Courtesy of CooperSurgical, Inc.)

Complications

Vaginal discharge and odor are common with prolonged pessary use and may indicate infection or epithelial abnormalities. Vaginal abrasions, granulation tissue, erosions, and ulcerations are the most common.[5,15] Management can include a "pessary holiday" in which the pessary is removed for 2–4 weeks to allow reepithelialization, as well as the use of vaginal estrogen cream if there are no contraindications. Rarely, vesicovaginal and rectovaginal fistulas, urinary retention, hydronephrosis, urosepsis, and small bowel entrapment have been reported. Another potential complication is pessary incarceration, most commonly seen with forgotten pessaries. Prolonged retention of a pessary without periodic cleaning can lead to contracture of the vaginal epithelium around the pessary leading to significant pain, infection, superficial epithelial erosions, urinary retention, and its sequelae, as well as the development of fistulous tracts to surrounding organs.[15–17] Patient and family education is imperative to ensure adequate management. Scheduling regular follow-up appointments even in the setting of self-management can aid in prevention and prompt treatment of these complications, and patients and caregivers should be encouraged to call with concerns or questions related to the pessary. Regular follow-up appointments allow patients to continue the use of incontinence pessaries for as long as they feel it is comfortable and effective.

Disposable Incontinence Devices

Disposable incontinence devices have been developed and marketed for use in recent years for women interested in the nonsurgical management of SUI in the setting of short periods of activity. Disposable incontinence devices come in varying sizes, and depending on the brand, sizing can be performed by the patient at home using a sizing kit or in the office similar to traditional incontinence pessaries. The Impressa bladder support device (Figure 3.6) is an FDA-approved over-the-counter disposable incontinence device marketed for up to 12 hours of use within a 24-hour period for the temporary management of SUI in women. This particular disposable incontinence device offers a sizing kit for at-home self-fitting and comes in three distinct sizes marketed for "low," "medium," and "high" levels of support. The sizing kit comes with two bladder supports of each size and has a retail value of $4.99, while single-size packs of 10 devices retail at $14.49 per package. The device is inserted into the vagina using a plastic applicator similar to that of a menstrual tampon, with a polyester and rayon string at the distal end that protrudes out of the vagina for self-removal. The device is constructed from medical-grade silicone and surrounded by a nonabsorbent polypropylene covering.

Data on the efficacy of disposable incontinence devices are limited. A recently presented crossover randomized controlled trial of women with SUI managed by Impressa and incontinence pessaries by Elshatanoufy et al.[18] at the American Urogynecologic Society 2018 Pelvic Floor Disorders Week showed no difference in pad weight, severity, or quality-of-life scores between the two devices. However, patients using the incontinence pessary reported a more significant improvement in SUI based on the Patient Global Impression of Improvement (PGI-I).[18] While disposable incontinence devices may provide convenience, ease of use and cost effectiveness should also be considered. Simpson et al.[19] performed a cost-utility analysis of nonsurgical treatments of SUI using the primary outcome of highest net monetary benefit (NMB) and a standard willingness-to-pay (WTP) threshold of $50,000 per quality-adjusted life-year (QALY) and found Impressa to have a higher NMB when compared to traditional pessaries. Although seemingly more cost effective at first glance, the authors went on to acknowledge that the model efficacy estimates for Impressa relied heavily on expert opinion and did not take treatment complications into account secondary to the paucity of well-designed studies assessing its use.[19] While disposable incontinence devices have a promising future in the nonsurgical management of SUI, further high-quality studies are necessary to evaluate their impact on patient quality of life, satisfaction, and efficacy in the treatment of SUI.

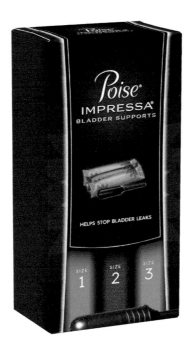

FIGURE 3.6   Impressa bladder support. (Courtesy of Kimberly-Clark, Corp.)

Conclusion

Incontinence pessaries are a reliable, first-line therapy for the treatment of SUI and should be considered in patients desiring nonsurgical management. This treatment has a low risk of adverse outcomes and, in the appropriate patient, can significantly improve quality of life. Incontinence pessaries, in addition to other behavioral and medical management options, should be discussed with all women seeking care for SUI.

REFERENCES

1. American College of Obstetricians and Gynecologists. Urinary incontinence in women. Practice Bulletin No. 155. *Obstet Gynecol.* 2015;126(5):66–81.
2. Luber KM. The definition, prevalence, and risk factors for stress urinary incontinence. *Rev Urol.* 2004;6(Suppl):S3–S9.
3. Dooley Y, Kenton K, Cao G et al. Urinary incontinence prevalence: Results from the National Health and Nutrition Examination Survey. *J Urol.* 2008;179(2):656–661.
4. Kenton K, Norton PA, Sirls LT et al. Retropubic versus transobturator midurethral slings for stress incontinence. *N Engl J Med.* 2010;362:2066–2076.

5. Al-Shaikh G, Syed S, Osman S, Bogis A, Al-Badr A. Pessary use in stress urinary incontinence: A review of advantages, complications, patient satisfaction, and quality of life. *Int J Womens Health.* 2018;10:195–201.
6. CooperSurgical. MILEX Pessary Reference Guide: Pessaries for Incontinence and Pelvic Organ Prolapse. 2011.
7. Nager CW, Richter HE, Nygaard I et al. Incontinence pessaries size, POPQ measures, and successful fitting. *Int Urogynecol J.* 2009;20(9):1023–1028.
8. Handa VL, Whitcomb E, Weidner AC et al. Sexual function before and after nonsurgical treatment of stress urinary incontinence. *Female Pelvic Med Reconstr Surg.* 2011;17(1):30–35.
9. Ding J, Chen C, Song XC, Zhang L, Deng M, Zhu L. Changes in prolapse and urinary symptoms after successful fitting of a ring pessary with support in women with advanced pelvic organ prolapse: A prospective study. *Urology.* 2016;87:70–75.
10. Clemons J, Aguilar V, Tillinghast T, Jackson ND, Myers DL. Patient satisfaction and changes in prolapse and urinary symptoms in women who are fitted successfully with a pessary for pelvic organ prolapse. *Am J Obstet Gynecol.* 2004;190(4):1025–1029.
11. Patel MS, Mellen C, O'Sullivan DM, Lasala CA. Pessary use and impact on quality of life and body image. *Female Pelvic Med Reconstr Surg.* 2011;17(6):298–301.
12. Jones KA, Harmanli O. Pessary use in pelvic organ prolapse and urinary incontinence. *Rev Obstet Gynecol.* 2010;3(1):3–9.
13. Kenton K, Barber M, Wang L et al. Pelvic floor symptoms improve similarly after pessary and behavioral treatment for stress incontinence. *Female Pelvic Med Reconstr Surg.* 2012;18(2):118–121.
14. Richter HE, Burgio KL, Brubaker L et al. A trial of continence pessary vs. behavioral therapy vs. combined therapy for stress incontinence. *Obstet Gynecol.* 2010;115(3):609–617.
15. O'Dell K, Atnip S. Pessary care: Follow-up and management of complications. *Urol Nurs.* 2012;32(3):126–136.
16. Arias BE, Ridgeway B, Barber MD. Complications of neglected vaginal pessaries: Case presentation and literature review. *Int Urogynecol J Pelvic Floor Dysfunct.* 2008;19(8):1173–1178.
17. Hanavadi S, Durham-Hall A, Oke T, Aston N. Forgotten vaginal pessary eroding into rectum. *Ann R Coll Surg Engl.* 2004;86(6):w18–w19.
18. Elshatanoufy S, Hicks B, Estanol M, Richardson D, Atiemo H, Luck A. American Urogynecologic Society Pelvic Floor Disorders Week abstracts, abstract 36. *Female Pelvic Med Reconstr Surg.* 2018;24(5S):S1–S17.
19. Simpson AN, Garbens A, Dossa F, Coyte PC, Baxter NN, McDermott CD. A cost-utility analysis of nonsurgical treatments for stress urinary incontinence in women. *Female Pelvic Med Reconstr Surg.* 2019;25(1):49–55.

4

Pessary Fitting

Hayley Barnes and Thythy Pham

CONTENTS

There is no standardized way to fit a pessary; most clinicians utilize a trial-and-error approach. In general, the goal is to fit the patient with a pessary that is comfortable while alleviating the patient's symptoms. The pessary should allow for voiding and defecatory functions and remain in place with activity or Valsalva. Prior to offering treatment with a pessary, a clinician should determine if a patient is an appropriate candidate. Contraindications to pessary use (outlined in Table 4.1) may include vaginal erosive disease, active infections of the vagina or pelvis, latex or silicone sensitivity, cancer of the lower genital tract including the cervix or vagina, or concern for noncompliance with follow-up.

In our practice, prior to fitting the pessary, we perform a comprehensive pelvic examination with an empty bladder in the dorsal lithotomy position to assess the postvoid urine residual and the stage of prolapse using a split speculum and the pelvic organ prolapse quantification (POPQ) system. A supine cough stress test is performed to determine the presence of stress urinary incontinence. If prolapse is present, a reduced cough stress test is also performed to assess for *de novo* stress urinary incontinence. Additionally, assessment for vaginal atrophy, narrowing, bleeding, or discharge is performed. We also assess the strength of the pelvic floor musculature, which is graded by the modified Oxford grading scale (Table 4.2). Finally, we assess for myofascial pain of the pelvic floor along the levator ani muscles and/or the obturator muscles. If pain is present, patients are asked to provide a pain level on a scale of 0 (pain free) to 10 (worst pain imaginable). Patients with significant myofascial pain may benefit from supervised pelvic floor physical therapy prior to use of a pessary, as they may find the pessary uncomfortable.

Several factors are considered in determining the type of pessary to trial. These factors include (1) the stage and type of prolapse present, (2) the sexual activity status of the patient, and (3) the patient's ability to manage the pessary. The latter requires the ability to reach into the vagina to remove the pessary;

TABLE 4.1

Contraindications to Pessary Use

Vaginal erosive disease
Active vaginal or pelvic infections
Latex or silicone sensitivity
Cancer of the lower genital tract
Undiagnosed vaginal bleeding
Severe vaginal atrophy
Concern for noncompliance with follow-up

TABLE 4.2

Modified Oxford Grading Scale for
Pelvic Floor Muscles

0	No muscle activity
1	Minor muscle "flicker"
2	Weak muscle activity without circular contraction
3	Moderate muscle contraction
4	Good muscle contraction
5	Strong muscle contraction

thus, the patient needs both hand strength and dexterity. We use the prolapse stage to guide selection of the pessary type and patient's vaginal introitus size, vaginal width, and vaginal length to guide the size of the pessary. To determine the most appropriate pessary size, we perform the following measurements. First, we estimate the size of the vaginal introitus by determining the number of fingerbreadths across the posterior fourchette, which is typically between 1 and 4 cm. Next, we determine the distance from the posterior fornix to the pubic symphysis using the examiner's pointer finger and thumb—this is roughly total vaginal length (TVL). Finally, we estimate the transverse vaginal width at the apex of the vagina with the index and middle fingers.

The most commonly used pessaries are ring, ring with support, Gellhorn, and donut pessaries.[1] A ring pessary or ring with support is a good first option for most patients. In a prospective study of 110 women, pessaries were successfully fitted in 74% of patients.[2] Of these, 96% were fitted with a ring pessary. Data suggest that in patients with a narrowed introitus (less than 1 to 2 fingerbreadths) or prolapse stages II or III, a ring pessary is more likely to be successful. In contrast, for patients with larger introituses or stage IV prolapse, they are more likely to benefit from a Gellhorn or space-occupying pessary.[3] The presence of vaginal shortening or narrowing will limit pessary selection to smaller sizes. In our practice, we typically start with a trial of a support pessary as these tend to be more comfortable and are easier for patients to manage. If a support pessary cannot be successfully fitted, trial and error is usually necessary to find the correct pessary size and shape for an individual patient.

Once we select a pessary type and size, we perform the fitting. The pessary is folded, and the leading edge is lubricated (Figures 4.1 and 4.2). The examiner's dominant hand holds the folded pessary, while the nondominant hand is used to separate the labia and introitus. The pessary (with lubrication on the leading edge at the clinician's discretion) is then introduced into the vagina over the

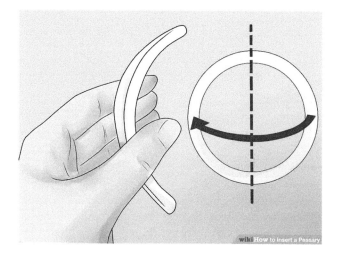

FIGURE 4.1 Folding the pessary (This series of illustrations is republished from wikiHow—https://www.wikihow.com/Insert-a-Pessary—under a Creative Commons License.)

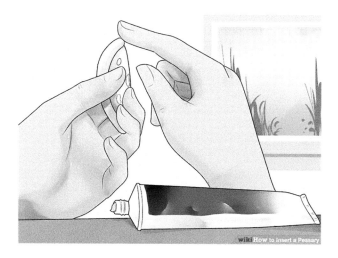

FIGURE 4.2 Lubricating the leading edge of the pessary.

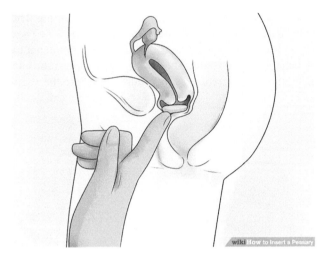

FIGURE 4.3   Pessary insertion.

perineum. Next, the index finger is used to position the pessary along an oblique axis with the anterior portion adjacent to the pubic symphysis and the posterior portion in the posterior vaginal fornix (Figure 4.3). We recommend that a pessary be sized so that the examiner's finger can comfortably fit around the circumference of the pessary. For those pessaries that only fold in one direction, the ring pessary should be turned one-quarter turn in either direction following placement to ensure that the foldable edge is not placed in front of the introitus. This will potentially limit spontaneous expulsion. If an incontinence ring or dish is used, the knob should be positioned under the mid-urethra.

Once the pessary is inserted and the correct position is ensured, we ask the patient to perform provocative maneuvers including standing, sitting, ambulation, coughing, and jumping (as able) to determine pessary retention and relief of symptoms. These measures also assist in the detection of the development of bothersome stress urinary incontinence. Patients are then escorted to the restroom to void and perform Valsalva while sitting on the toilet to ensure voiding ability and check for pessary expulsion. This process is repeated with additional pessary sizes and/or types until determination of the optimal pessary is made. The goal is that the resultant pessary choice is both comfortable for the patient and alleviates her symptoms.

Ring pessaries with and without support and continence rings and dishes are the easiest to fold, insert, and remove. Gellhorn and cube pessaries are more difficult to insert and remove as they are held in place by significant space occupation and suction, though they offer strong support. The suction of these pessaries needs to be broken before removal. A Shaatz pessary is fitted with the convex portion placed anteriorly. A Gellhorn pessary is fitted by folding of the disc when possible with the stem folded down for ease of insertion. The stem will be directed caudally (pointing out), and it should be possible to pass a finger between the disc and the vaginal side wall. If the vagina is foreshortened and the patient notices the stem protruding from the introitus, a short-stem Gellhorn pessary may be a better option in her specific circumstance. Because of its shape and mechanism of action (suction), a cube pessary does not need to be as large as the width of the vagina. Insertion of a cube pessary involves compressing the edge that is introduced into the vaginal opening and pushing it up and back. Donut pessaries also require compression for insertion.

At the conclusion of the pessary fitting visit, the patient is informed of potential complications of pessary use, including urinary retention, defecatory dysfunction, vaginal bleeding, or erosions, and is instructed to call with the development of any concerning symptoms. We prescribe biweekly vaginal estrogen for women with symptoms or signs of concurrent vaginal atrophy. Patients then are asked to schedule a 2- to 4-week follow-up appointment and instructed to monitor their symptoms during that time period.

At the follow-up appointment, a directed history is obtained including the relief or persistence of vaginal bulge or pressure symptoms, discomfort, expulsion, voiding or defecatory dysfunction, development of stress urinary incontinence, and vaginal bleeding or discharge. The pessary is then removed. Once removed, the pessary should be washed with soap and water. The perforation of the Gellhorn and Shaatz pessaries can be cleansed with a cytobrush or small cotton swab. The vaginal epithelium is examined for the presence of bleeding, abrasions, or erosions. If the vaginal exam is reassuring and the patient reports satisfaction with the trial of the pessary, she is then taught to remove, clean, and reinsert the pessary independently. We recommend removal once or twice per month in patients able to perform home pessary maintenance.

After the initial follow-up, continued follow-up is recommended at 6- and 12-month intervals at the discretion of the provider. If the patient is unable to remove and insert her pessary independently, she is instructed to return for removal and cleaning by a provider at approximately 3-month intervals. Maintenance of pessary care by a provider rather than the patient is often required with Gellhorn, cube, or donut pessaries.

Some pessaries may be difficult to remove. The Gellhorn pessary is easier to remove when the provider uses a ring or packing forceps on the base of the stem to apply outward traction. Simultaneous with the outward traction, the clinician inserts a gloved, lubricated (usually index) finger of the contralateral hand to reach just beyond the disc of the pessary. Once the distal interphalangeal joint is around the disc, it can be folded against the stem. Once folded, the index finger and ring forceps are gently pulled outward and downward to remove the pessary as painlessly as possible. A cube pessary requires removal and cleaning more often than every 3 months, because a greater amount of discharge can be accumulated within the suction cups, though some cube pessaries have drainage holes. The frequency of cleaning required for a cube pessary will vary among patients, from every few days to every month.

On each follow-up visit, proper placement of the pessary and alleviation of symptoms are assessed. Because pessaries are fit by a process of trial and error, it is sometimes necessary to change the pessary size or type after the initial fitting. During the follow-up visit, the integrity of the pessary and the health of the patient's vaginal tissue are also checked for irritation, pressure sores, ulcerations, and estrogen status. Women can be sexually active with the ring or Shaatz pessary in place. A cube, donut, or Gellhorn pessary must generally be removed before intercourse.

Despite best efforts, a trial of pessary is unsuccessful in certain patients. Approximately a quarter of patients cannot be fitted with a pessary, while half discontinue pessary use shortly after being successfully fitted.[2,4,5] Prior research has identified patient factors that are associated with an increased risk of pessary fitting failure. These factors can be divided into patient demographics, surgical history, and physical exam findings. When considering a patient's demographics, data show that age younger than 65 years, tobacco use, and obesity may contribute to a lower success rate.[6] Characteristics that were associated with continued pessary use after 1 year were older age and poor surgical risk.[3] Geoffrion et al. propose that younger women more often prefer surgery over conservative management for prolapse treatment and suggest that smokers may have more difficulty with pessary wear due to a thinner vaginal mucosal layer. A history of prior hysterectomy (non-route specific) and pelvic organ prolapse repair have also been proven to influence the short-term success of pessary therapy.[7,8] Initial pelvic exam findings also suggest a higher rate of failed pessary trials. These include a wide vaginal introitus (greater than 4 fingerbreadths), short total vaginal length (less than 6 cm), a genital hiatus/total vaginal length ratio of less than 0.8, lower grades of prolapse, and current rectocele.[3,9] One should note that the measurement of the vaginal introitus is not part of the POPQ system. A wide vaginal introitus is indicative of separation of the bulbocavernosus muscle from the perineal body, which in turn allows for distension of the introitus and makes pessary retention more difficult. In our experience, women with short vaginal lengths, if able to be fitted with a pessary, will require smaller pessaries, and women with wide vaginal openings will require larger pessaries to allow for retention. Women with higher grades of prolapse (III–IV) are more likely to require a space-filling pessary such as a Gellhorn.

Problems that may arise following a successful pessary fitting are as follows. Patients may complain of vaginal discharge or odor that is often precipitated by a foreign-body reaction to the pessary. We suggest ruling out acute vaginitis. A topical cream such as Trimo-San cream (Cooper Surgical) or Replens may decrease odor and discharge. If vaginal bleeding occurs, we recommend ruling out a vaginal abrasion or ulcer. If either is present, we would remove the pessary for a period of 2–4 weeks and prescribe vaginal estrogen to allow the area to heal. Resolution of erosions may also occur without local estrogen.[10] We also consider a smaller pessary size to prevent bleeding caused by friction. It is important to rule out other sources of bleeding such as uterine or cervical etiology. If the patient experiences pain or urinary or fecal retention, her pessary may be too large, and we suggest downsizing. Finally, upsizing of the pessary may be needed if the pessary is frequently expelled. This can be averted by preventing constipation and minimizing straining in general. Major complications, such as fistula and incarcerated pessaries, are uncommon—91% were related to neglected pessaries.[11] Therefore, the importance of continued and diligent follow-up in a patient using a pessary is stressed.

Conclusion

Pessary fitting can be accomplished with minimal ease in a vast majority of patients with basic providers' training. Optimization of pessary fitting can be achieved with consideration of patient's anatomy, diagnoses and ability to perform self-maintenance. The best fit pessary is one that is comfortable and provides relief of the patient's symptoms.

REFERENCES

1. Cundiff GW, Weidner AC, Visco AG, Bump RC, Addison WA. A survey of pessary use by members of the American Urogynecologic Society. *Obstet Gynecol.* 2000;95(6 Pt 1):931–935.
2. Wu V, Farrell SA, Baskett TF, Flowerdew G. A simplified protocol for pessary management. *Obstet Gynecol.* 1997;90(6):990–994.
3. Clemons JL, Aguilar VC, Tillinghast TA, Jackson ND, Myers DL. Risk factors associated with an unsuccessful pessary fitting trial in women with pelvic organ prolapse. *Am J Obstet Gynecol.* 2004;190(2):345–350.
4. Sulak PJ, Kuehl TJ, Shull BL. Vaginal pessaries and their use in pelvic relaxation. *J Reprod Med.* 1993;38(12):919–923.
5. Myers DL, LaSala CA, Murphy JA. Double pessary use in grade 4 uterine and vaginal prolapse. *Obstet Gynecol.* 1998;91(6):1019–1020.
6. Geoffrion R, Zhang T, Lee T, Cundiff GW. Clinical characteristics associated with unsuccessful pessary fitting outcomes. *Female Pelvic Med Reconstr Surg.* 2013;19(6):339–345.
7. Mutone MF, Terry C, Hale DS, Benson JT. Factors which influence the short-term success of pessary management of pelvic organ prolapse. *Am J Obstet Gynecol.* 2005;193(1):89–94.
8. Nemeth Z, Farkas N, Farkas B. Is hysterectomy or prior reconstructive surgery associated with unsuccessful initial trial of pessary fitting in women with symptomatic pelvic organ prolapse? *Int Urogynecol J.* 2017;28(5):757–761.

9. Yamada T, Matsubara S. Rectocoele, but not cystocoele, may predict unsuccessful pessary fitting. *J Obstet Gynaecol.* 2011;31(5):441–442.

10. Hanson LA, Schulz JA, Flood CG, Cooley B, Tam F. Vaginal pessaries in managing women with pelvic organ prolapse and urinary incontinence: Patient characteristics and factors contributing to success. *Int Urogynecol J Pelvic Floor Dysfunct.* 2006;17(2):155–159.

11. Arias BE, Ridgeway B, Barber MD. Complications of neglected vaginal pessaries: Case presentation and literature review. *Int Urogynecol J Pelvic Floor Dysfunct.* 2008;19(8):1173–1178.

5

Pessary Care

Marko J. Jachtorowycz

CONTENTS

Pelvic organ prolapse is a quality-of-life disorder that affects a significant portion of the female population. A pessary is a useful tool at the clinician's disposal for the treatment of symptoms brought on by pelvic organ prolapse. It can also help to manage some urinary symptoms such as stress urinary incontinence related to urethral hypermobility and/or urinary outflow obstruction related to pelvic organ prolapse. In addition, it can alleviate anorectal symptoms associated with a rectocele.[1] A properly fitted pessary can significantly improve the quality of life for those afflicted with symptoms related to pelvic organ prolapse.[2,3] Care and follow-up for patients wearing a pessary require a commitment by the patient (and in some cases her care providers) as well as customization of follow-up recommendations from the treating clinician.

The pessary can serve as an interim or a long-term management solution for the spectrum of symptoms caused by pelvic support defects. Use of a pessary for all these reasons requires the managing clinician to guide and oversee each patient's care and use of a pessary. There are no absolute guidelines for follow-up and care of the pessary, and practices vary widely among clinicians.[4,5] Each pessary wearer will adapt to the presence of the device uniquely. Many women may develop symptoms of discharge or odor in relatively short time frames, while others may be free of troubling symptoms for long periods of time. The guiding principle underlying customization of follow-up is improved quality of life through relief of symptoms.

The introduction of a pessary into the lower genital tract impacts the vagina in several ways. A pessary placed in the vagina will contact and put a degree of pressure on the genital mucosa. In addition, the pessary is a foreign body that will impact the vaginal microenvironment.[6] An understanding of the uniqueness of the vaginal microenvironment is key to successful care and management of a pessary. The vagina is not a sterile environment and is home to numerous species of bacteria as well as several species of fungi. Among the bacteria are anaerobes and aerobes, lactose splitters, and gram-negative species. In the typical vaginal microenvironment, the number of anaerobes is kept in check by the relatively acidic environment created by lactose splitting bacteria.[7] Alterations in that microenvironment can result in the proliferation of anaerobic bacteria that can give rise to clinical symptoms such as discharge, odor, and genital irritation.

Complications of pessary use may also include the formation of vesicovaginal or rectovaginal fistulas.[8] Pessary incarceration requiring either morcellation of the pessary or removal under anesthesia can occur with pessary neglect. These complications are generally very uncommon and rarely occur in patients who are appropriately followed. Proper follow-up and ongoing care and management are key to successful pessary use.

Two-thirds of women with symptoms related to pelvic organ prolapse can be successfully managed with a pessary.[9] Continuation rates of pessary use are generally high.

Initiating Pessary Use

There are five stages of initiation for pessary use:

1. Initial fitting
2. Upright stress test
3. Ambulation and voiding test
4. Initial trial
5. Prolonged trial

When the candidate pessary user successfully negotiates these stages, she is ready to transition to ongoing care and maintenance.

Initial Fitting (Beginning of the First Visit)

It is essential to assess the potential for success when a pessary is first fitted. Once the appropriate geometry and the right size are selected, the clinician should determine the pessary wearer's comfort when the pessary is in place. If the patient is comfortable with the pessary in place and reports no pain or excessive pressure, she is ready to progress to the next phase of the initial trial.

Upright Stress Test (Middle of the First Visit)

With the pessary in place, the patient should be asked to stand and, if possible, separate and bend her knees while the clinician looks at the vaginal introitus directly or with a strategically placed hand mirror. This initial "stress test" will provide a glimpse as to how well the pessary is seated in the lower genital tract. It will also provide an idea of the amount of movement (displacement) that occurs with increases in abdominal pressure. Feedback on how the pessary feels when in place should be elicited from the wearer. The sensation of the "presence" of an object in the lower genital tract is normal. Pain is an indication that the selected pessary may be too large or may not be the right shape. A pessary should be "big enough to do the job (of providing support), but small enough to be comfortable." Physical limitations of some patients may preclude the ability to perform this phase of testing. In the absence of the ability to do this, the clinician may choose to determine how much traction it takes to dislodge the pessary with the patient in the supine position or in the upright position (if she can be helped to stand by an office assistant, caregiver, or family member).

For patients being managed for stress urinary incontinence, this phase of testing provides an opportunity to assess the degree to which the presence of the pessary reduces or eliminates urine loss. While upright, the patient should be asked to cough or to perform the Valsalva maneuver as the clinician observes for the adequacy of support and any urine loss. For patients being managed with a pessary for genital prolapse, this will help determine whether a reduction of genital prolapse will uncover the symptom of stress urinary incontinence.

If the pessary does not dislodge and fall out during the upright stress test, the wearer is ready to progress to the initial ambulation and voiding test.

Ambulation and Voiding Test and Initial Trial (End of the First Visit)

After fitting and initial anatomic stress testing of the pessary, the wearer should be encouraged to ambulate within the office or clinic for a brief time and void. Any early shift of the pessary to an uncomfortable location within the genital tract should prompt a refitting. The wearer should be encouraged to void. If there is difficulty with initiating a urinary stream or if there is retention or dysuria, the pessary should be refitted or replaced with another size and/or shape. If the ambulation and voiding trial uncovers no issues, the wearer is ready for an initial trial with the pessary and may leave the office or clinic with planned follow-up in a short interval of time (e.g., a few days to a month).

Assessment of Initial Trial (Begins at the End of the First Visit and Runs through the Second Visit)

After initial success in the office, the pessary wearer is ready for an "initial trial." She may be discharged from the office or clinic and should be seen for follow-up in a short interval of time, but ideally no later than 30 days after the initial visit. At the follow-up visit, the patient is assessed for the appearance, exacerbation, evolution, resolution, or alleviation of any urinary symptoms. She should be queried regarding pain, discharge, odor, genital bleeding, or pressure symptoms.

At the initial portion of the second examination (if the wearer's physical ability permits), the patient should again be examined in the upright position with the genital tract viewed directly or with the assistance of a hand mirror. The position of the pessary should be assessed (if any portion of the pessary is visible). The clinician may choose to gently apply downward pressure on the pessary to ascertain the stability of its position.

An examination in the dorsal lithotomy position is conducted at the first follow-up visit. The pessary should be removed, cleaned, and inspected. A speculum exam is performed, and the lower genital tract inspected for erosions or ulcerations of the vaginal mucosa. The anatomic location of any erosion(s) should be noted and factored into any decision involving pessary change (size or shape). If a pessary change is required, the same steps outlined earlier (initial stress test, ambulation and voiding trial, and initial field test) should be repeated.

If no ulcerations or erosions are identified, the pessary wearer is ready to proceed to the prolonged trial and should return in a longer interval of time for a rexamination. A useful guide is to double the time used for the initial trial. However, if that was a very short interval, it is reasonable to allow a month for follow-up. If the initial trial was for up to 30 days, then one could move to a 2-month prolonged trial.

At this time, the clinician and the patient should discuss and explore the specifics of ongoing management. In general terms, the pessary should be removed and cleaned regularly. Some women may choose to learn how to remove and replace the pessary. Those who are candidates for self-guided removal and replacement should be trained on the steps of placement, removal, and replacement in the office by a qualified provider, either a physician or a nonphysician clinician.

Most women who choose to remove and replace the pessary on their own can do so in the supine position on a bed or sofa with legs separated. Others may prefer to stand with one leg in a higher position (foot resting on a step or bathtub rim). Once self-placement and removal proficiency is confirmed, the patient is ready for a prolonged trial. She should practice removing and replacing the pessary and return for a follow-up visit and examination.

Many wearers will be unable to remove and replace their pessary for a variety of reasons ranging from physical impairment to individual preference. Pessary care for these individuals will be entirely in the hands of their clinician and will require more frequent visits. Once the follow-up regimen has been decided, the patient is ready for a prolonged trial and should return in 30–90 days for a follow-up visit and examination.

Prolonged Trial (Starts at the End of the Second Visit and Runs through the Start of the Third Visit)

After the initial trial, pessary wearers should return after a prolonged trial of 30–90 days. This visit is similar to the visit after the initial trial. The patient should be assessed through examination in the upright and supine positions. Pessary removal, cleaning, and inspection are done. The genital tract is examined and evaluated for erosions or ulcerations. If the exam is negative for any of these issues, the wearer is ready to move onto the care and maintenance phase of pessary use. (See Table 5.1.)

TABLE 5.1

Pessary Treatment

Phase of Pessary Initiation	Location	Timing
Initial fitting	Office or clinic	
Upright stress test	Office or clinic	
Ambulation and void test	Office or clinic	
Initial trial	Home/ambulatory	
Clinical exam after initial trial	Office or clinic	1–30 days after fitting
Prolonged trial	Home/ambulatory	
Clinical exam after prolonged trial	Office or clinic	30–90 days after fitting
Ongoing pessary use	Home/ambulatory	
Maintenance visits	Office or clinic	30-day to annual intervals[a]

[a] Individualized to each wearer's ability or inability to remove, clean, and place.

Ongoing Pessary Care and Maintenance Visits

Once the prolonged trial has been successful, pessary wearers must be followed on an ongoing basis. Women who can remove and replace their pessaries are generally advised to remove their pessaries regularly. The definition of "regular" varies. There are no well-established criteria for the frequency of removal and cleaning. Many users will customize their removal schedule. Some will remove their pessary nightly or weekly, while others will remove their pessary monthly or even less often. It is recommended that users keep their pessaries in place for a maximum of 90 days, though intervals of twice that long have not been associated with any particular complications.[8,9] Follow-up for women who remove and clean their pessaries should be every 6–12 months.

For pessary users who do not remove and clean their pessaries, follow-up intervals of 90 days have been recommended. Adhering to such a schedule is an appropriate initial plan. Follow-up intervals can be individualized for each wearer.[10] Rarely would such a patient be allowed to spread out visits to only annual follow-up. Usually, the interval is self-determined by the initiation of any discharge or odor that develops. Such symptoms can be minimized by choosing an interval shorter than when such symptoms develop. At each visit, the clinician should carefully inspect the pessary and assess its overall condition as it is cleaned with soap and water.

Individualizing Follow-Up and Managing Pessary-Related Symptoms

Factors that will affect success and satisfaction with the pessary include discharge and odor as well as pain with placement and removal of the pessary.

The presence of a foreign body in an environment that is not sterile has the potential to lead to the proliferation of certain bacteria. In the case of the pessary in the vaginal microenvironment, the adherence of aerobic and anaerobic bacteria to the pessary and the subsequent proliferation of these organisms will alter the general bacterial balance of the lower genital tract. This proliferation of aerobic and anaerobic bacteria (particularly the anaerobes) will create a discharge and very often an odor. Wearers who regularly change their pessary can combat this with more frequent removal and cleaning. Pessary users who do not remove and clean their pessaries will be more likely to develop these symptoms. There are several options for alleviating the symptoms of odor and discharge. The first of these is more frequent removal and cleaning of the pessary requiring visit adjustment to a schedule with sufficient frequency to minimize or eliminate the onset of these symptoms. Alternatively, the user may be offered another option to reduce or manage pessary-related odor and discharge.

The use of oxyquinoline sulfate and sodium lauryl sulfate jelly (Trimo-San) twice weekly is an accepted method to restore vaginal acidity and reduce the proliferation of bacteria in the vagina.[11] This over-the-counter agent has few side effects and represents a safe, nonhormonal method for control of pessary-related odor and discharge.

The addition of local estrogen to the pessary-containing vaginal microenvironment is another option for management of discharge and odor.[12] The local effect of estrogen promotes increased vascularity, increased mucus production from the vaginal epithelium, and proliferation of lactic acid–producing microbes. Topical estrogen will restore the acidic pH of the vaginal microenvironment and reduce the proliferation of anaerobic bacteria and thus reduce the accompanying odor and discharge. Local estrogen will also thicken the genital mucosa increasing its resistance to erosion, abrasion, and ulceration from the pessary. Though the systemic absorption of estrogens from locally administered estrogen is minimal, contraindications to estrogen use in the wearer's history need to be considered. Local estrogen may be used judiciously in patients with a personal history of thromboembolic disease and those with a personal history of an estrogen-dependent malignancy (most commonly breast cancer and endometrial cancer).

There is controversy as to the safety of vaginal estrogen in patients who have a personal history of endometrial or breast cancer. The general guideline that most clinicians follow is to initially consider local estrogen in the same manner as a systemic replacement and consider the contraindications identical. However, given the minimal systemic absorption of local estrogen, its use in certain circumstances for breast cancer and endometrial cancer survivors can be individualized. In the case of breast cancer, the estrogen receptor status, degree of spread at the time of diagnosis, as well as time since treatment will affect the decision regarding local estrogen use. In the case of endometrial cancer, the degree of spread at diagnosis, the degree of differentiation (grade) of the tumor, as well as time since treatment will have a bearing on the decision to use local estrogen. The decision may also be made in consultation with the treating oncologist.

Clinicians should consider spacing visit frequency differently in patients wearing a pessary. Another option for patients who develop problematic discharge or odor is periodic use of a vaginal douche. A weak vinegar douche can cleanse the secretions while also restoring vaginal acidity. This may allow an increased interval between visits, especially in cases where the development of odor or discharge is the only complaint and the wearer has achieved otherwise excellent symptom relief with the pessary.

Pain on placement and removal of the pessary may be managed with local anesthetic cream or gel applied 5 minutes before planned pessary change.[13]

Special Situations

Vaginal Ulcer

The symptoms of vaginal bleeding in a pessary wearer should prompt assessment for a vaginal ulcer resulting from pressure necrosis on the mucosa. Ulcers that do not bleed may be identified on routine follow-up exam. If an ulcer is identified, the pessary should not be replaced and the wearer should be advised to take a 2-week "pessary holiday" (with use of local estrogen cream if not contraindicated). The genital tract should be reassessed after the 2 weeks. If the ulcer or ulcers has/have healed, it is appropriate to restart pessary use. This situation will likely require a pessary refitting with a change in size or geometry.

Incarcerated Pessary

The forgotten pessary presents the treating clinician with the responsibility of safe removal and proper assessment of the wearer's genital tract. These patients will often be referred for evaluation of a discharge (which may be foul smelling) or with genital bleeding. The clinician should gently examine (to the degree possible) the genital tract with the pessary in place to ascertain its mobility.[14] If there are no unusual scar attachments and the pessary is mobile, removal with lubricant (and local anesthetic gel if needed) and gentle traction can be attempted. If this maneuver is not successful, it may be necessary to reattempt pessary removal with the patient under sedation or anesthesia.

If unusual or heavy scarring is identified, it may be necessary to morcellate the pessary. This can be accomplished with heavy scissors or a small wire cutter. Once the pessary is divided, it can be removed piecemeal without risk of injury to the mucosa of the lower genital tract. After removal by morcellation, the genital tract should be carefully examined. Any ulcers should be treated appropriately (if local estrogen is an option) and the patient should be followed carefully over a period of weeks. Once the genital tract has healed, pessary refitting (if appropriate) can be considered.

Magnetic Resonance Imaging

Pessary wearers who require magnetic resonance imaging (MRI) will be required to complete a questionnaire regarding any metallic implants or prostheses. A variety of pessary shapes exist, the majority of which do not contain metal. There are some that may contain metallic elements (such as a spring). These pessaries may cause artifacts or may pose safety risks for patients undergoing MRI scans. When a pessary wearer is scheduled to undergo an MRI, the managing clinician should check the type of pessary and determine whether it contains metal. There are various databases that list implants and medical devices and categorize them for MRI compatibility (an example of a searchable database of compatible MRI safe devices is accessible at http://www.mrisafety.com/TMDL_list.php).[15] Such a database can be queried before the planned imaging procedure. If the pessary in question is not listed as safe or if there is any question, it should be removed before the study.

Colonoscopy

Pessary wearers often inquire as to the disposition of their pessary during a colonoscopy. In general, a vaginal pessary will not interfere with colonoscopy. The endoscopist should be made aware of its presence, as at colonoscopy a pessary may create an extrinsic compression visible in the distal portion of the rectum.

Airport Security

Security screening at modern airports includes either a metal detector scan or a body image scan. Most use millimeter wave advanced imaging technology (AIT) and walk-through metal detectors to screen passengers. There have been no reports of pessary-related issues at airport safety checkpoints. It is advisable, however, that pessary wearers who travel by air be prepared for the possibility that a vaginal pessary may image on millimeter wave scanner or trigger the metal detector. Pessary wearers should be made aware of this possibility. If the wearer can remove her pessary, she should be advised to do so before entering airport security screening. For those who cannot remove their pessary, the best practice advice would be to follow the established precedent set for individuals with implanted prosthetic devices.[16] The patient is provided a letter signed by the treating clinician indicating the condition and the existence of an implant that may image on scanning or may be discovered by a metal detector.[17] In the United States, the pessary-wearing passenger may obtain a notification card from the Transportation Safety Administration,[18] which is presented at the time of screening.

Pessary Deterioration

Most pessaries have a long service life. However, continuous exposure to the bacterial milieu of the lower genital tract may lead to the formation of an adherent film or discharge that may discolor the pessary (Figure 5.1). Discoloration in and of itself is usually not a reason for pessary replacement with a new device, though some users may choose to procure a new device.

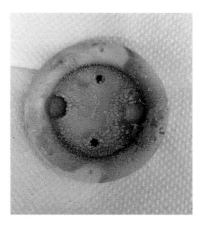

FIGURE 5.1 Example of pessary deterioration with discoloration and surface irregularities. (Photo credit: Alissa Roberts, APN.)

With placement and removal, some of the points of flexion (in the case of some shapes) of the pessary may lead to interruptions in the integrity of the device's surface and potentially create edges that may not be smooth. In rare cases, metallic portions of a pessary may become exposed. A pessary, which is damaged from use needs to be replaced.

Conclusion

Pessary management of genital prolapse and urinary incontinence represents an effective and nonsurgical solution that can be offered to any woman with genital prolapse who is either unable to undergo surgical repair or prefers to manage her symptoms without surgery. It has also been shown to improve anorectal symptoms and to generally improve quality of life. Pessary use requires commitment to care and follow-up by the patient and/or caregiver. In addition, it requires the treating clinician to appropriately assess progress with the pessary and recommend the timing of interval visits, which are individualized to each patient.

REFERENCES

1. Brazell H, Patel M, O'Sullivan D, Mellen C, LaSala C. The impact of pessary use on bowel symptoms. *Female Pelvic Med Reconstr Surg.* 2014;20(2):95–98.
2. Manchana T, Bunyavejchevin S. Impact on quality of life after ring pessary use for pelvic organ prolapse. *Int Urogynecol J.* 2012;23(7):873–877.

3. Coelho S, Marangoni-Junior M, Brito L, Castro E, Juliato C. Quality of life and vaginal symptoms of postmenopausal women using pessary for pelvic organ prolapse: A prospective study. *Rev Assoc Méd Bras.* 2018;64(12):1103–1107.

4. Dueñas J, Miceli A. Effectiveness of a continuous-use ring-shaped vaginal pessary without support for advanced pelvic organ prolapse in postmenopausal women. *Int Urogynecol J.* 2018;29(11):1629–1636.

5. Khaja A, Freeman R. How often should shelf/Gellhorn pessaries be changed? A survey of IUGA urogynaecologists. *Int Urogynecol J.* 2014;25(7):941–946.

6. Collins S, Beigi R, Mellen C, O'Sullivan D, Tulikangas P. The effect of pessaries on the vaginal microenvironment. *Am J Obstet Gynecol.* 2015;212(1):60.e1–60.e6.

7. Yoshimura K, Morotomi N, Fukuda K, Hachisuga T, Taniguchi H. Effects of pelvic organ prolapse ring pessary therapy on intravaginal microbial flora. *Int Urogynecol J.* 2016;27(2):219–227.

8. Arias B, Ridgeway B, Barber M. Complications of neglected vaginal pessaries: Case presentation and literature review. *Int Urogynecol J Pelvic Floor Dysfunct.* 2008;19(8):1173–1178.

9. Ramsay S, Tu L, Tannenbaum C. Natural history of pessary use in women aged 65–74 versus 75 years and older with pelvic organ prolapse: A 12-year study. *Int Urogynecol J.* 2016;27(8):1201–1207.

10. O'Dell K, Atnip S, Hooper G, Leung K. Pessary practices of nurse-providers in the United States. *Female Pelvic Med Reconstr Surg.* 2016;22(4):261–266.

11. Meriwether K, Rogers R, Craig E, Peterson S, Gutman R, Iglesia C. The effect of hydroxyquinoline-based gel on pessary-associated bacterial vaginosis: A multicenter randomized controlled trial. *Am J Obstet Gynecol.* 2015;213(5):729. e1–729.e9.

12. Dessie S, Armstrong K, Modest A, Hacker M, Hota L. Effect of vaginal estrogen on pessary use. *Int Urogynecol J.* 2016;27(9):1423–1429.

13. Taege S, Adams W, Mueller E, Brubaker L, Fitzgerald C, Brincat C. Anesthetic cream use during office pessary removal and replacement: A randomized controlled trial. *Obstet Gynecol.* 2017;130(1):190–197.

14. Poma, PA. Management of incarcerated vaginal pessaries. *J Am Geriatr Soc.* 1981 Jul;29(7):325–327.

15. http://www.mrisafety.com/TMDL_list.php, MRI Safety, The LIST and Safety Topics, Accessed September 6, 2019.

16. Ali E, Kosuge D, MacDowell A. The need for an implant identification card at airport security check. *Clin Orthop Surg.* 2017;9(2):153–159.

17. Asch M, Liu D, Mawdsley G. Detection of implanted metallic devices by airport security. *J Vasc Interv Radiol.* 1997 Nov–Dec;8(6):1011–1014.

18. https://www.tsa.gov/sites/default/files/disability_notification_card_508.pdf, TSA Notification Card: Individuals with Disabilities and Medical Conditions, Accessed September 6, 2019.

6

Outcomes of Pessary Use

Soo Kwon and Kara Griffith

CONTENTS

Throughout history, various forms of pessaries have been used to manage pelvic organ prolapse and/or stress urinary incontinence. In the past, a limited number of pessary options and the resultant problems that they produced led to nonuse or discontinuation of the use of a pessary in many patients. Today, however, we have multiple types of pessaries that allow for a more anatomic and comfortable fit for patients depending on their vaginal structure and symptomatology.

Pessaries serve as a nonsurgical management option. They are ideal for patients who desire nonsurgical management of their problem or for those who are not appropriate surgical candidates, such as the medically compromised elderly and all those patients with other medical comorbidities that make surgery high risk. With minimal side effects and rare complications, the pessary remains an effective option for the management of prolapse and incontinence for most patients (Table 6.1).

Benefits of Pessary Use

Not only can pessaries manage prolapse and incontinence symptoms, but they can also be used to provide diagnostic and predictive information regarding the effects of surgical management for prolapse and/or incontinence. For example, a prolapse reduction trial with a pessary in patients with symptomatic anterior vaginal wall prolapse and urinary retention has been shown to demonstrate good sensitivity, specificity, and positive predictive value for postoperative voiding function.[1]

Pessaries have also been shown to have a positive effect on patients' quality of life, body image, anxiety, and bowel function. Although one reason for the discontinuation of a pessary is expulsion, if properly fitted, the continuation rate for pessary use as management for incontinence and/or prolapse has been reported to be as high as 90%.[2]

Efficacy for Pelvic Organ Prolapse

Although significantly higher patient satisfaction was achieved with surgical management, Sung et al. found that those who continued pessary use had a high goal achievement rating with a 70% improvement in all symptom categories and a 79.3% improvement in prolapse goals as demonstrated by the Patient-Reported Outcomes Measurement Information System (PROMIS) questionnaires. However, 40% discontinued the pessary or crossed over to a surgical option. For women who were dissatisfied and discontinued pessary use, reasons included discomfort, continued bulge symptoms, urinary symptoms, bowel symptoms, inconvenience, and vaginal discharge.[3] Clemons et al. further demonstrated this in their study. Of those successfully fitted for a pessary, satisfaction occurred in 77%–92% of women. In addition, there was a significant decrease in bulge symptoms and splinting at 2 months.[4]

Efficacy for Stress Urinary Incontinence

Incontinence pessaries serve as a nonsurgical management option and are inserted into the vagina to provide support to the urethrovesical junction and anterior vaginal wall. By providing compression to the urethra against the pubic symphysis, urinary incontinence is ameliorated when intra-abdominal pressure is increased.[5,6] An incontinence pessary similarly provides support to a mid-urethral sling while avoiding a surgical procedure. Various pessaries of this nature are available, including the anti-incontinence ring with and without support, the anti-incontinence dish, and the Uresta incontinence pessary. A retrospective chart review of 100 patients demonstrated a 59% continued pessary use at 11 months and reported a resolution or improvement in incontinence.[7]

When a pessary is used for the treatment of stress urinary incontinence, it can be inserted on either a continuous or intermittent basis (e.g., during incontinence-provoking activities like exercise). The Ambulatory Treatments for Leakage Associated with Stress (ATLAS) trial compared the use of pessary alone, combined pessary with behavioral therapy, and behavioral therapy alone at 3, 6, and 12 months.[8] This study used the Urogenital Distress

Inventory–Stress Incontinence category of the Pelvic Floor Distress Inventory and Patient Global Impression of Improvement to assess treatment efficacy. The results at 3 months were different than at 12 months. At 3 months, the patients were less satisfied with pessary management than with behavioral therapy (63% in the pessary group versus 75% in the behavioral group). Although both groups reported an improvement in urinary incontinence, 49% of those in the behavioral group were without bothersome symptoms compared to 33% in the pessary group. At 12 months, success rates had declined in both the pessary and behavioral groups, and these differences were no longer significant (Table 6.1).

Effects on Quality of Life and Sexual Function

Not only do pessaries provide good objective outcomes for the management of both prolapse and urinary incontinence, but pessaries have also been shown to improve quality of life, body image scores, and sexual function (Table 6.2). Quality of life and depressive symptom scores improve with pessary use. However, there is less improvement seen in patients with depressive symptoms.[9] Pessaries in combination with exercise therapy can also improve quality of life compared to exercise therapy alone.[10] Although continued follow-up is required for all pessary users, there is no difference in the impact on the quality of life in those who provide self-care for pessary maintenance and those who require provider maintenance.[11]

Whether or not a patient is sexually active does have an impact on which pessary should be used. Although sexually active women are overall more likely to continue a pessary long term regardless of the indication for placement, some pessaries require removal before intercourse, such as the space-occupying pessaries (e.g., cube, Gellhorn, and donut pessaries).[12] In a secondary analysis of a randomized controlled trial of new pessary users, satisfaction with pessary use was associated with improved sexual function scores and improved modified body image scale scores. In this analysis, 70% of patients removed their pessary before intercourse, with 53% stating their partner preferred removal.[13]

Complications and Side Effects Associated with Pessary Use

Complications resulting from pessary use are typically minor, resulting in little or no harm. Major complications are rare. The overall complication rate ranges from 15% to 73%.[14,15] Regardless of these complications, the majority of patients are satisfied with pessary use and choose to continue its use. The most common complication resulting from pessary use is an increase in vaginal discharge. Pessary expulsion, significant vaginal erosion, bleeding, irritation, and occult incontinence are not uncommon. Significant

TABLE 6.1

Outcomes of Pessary Use for Incontinence and Prolapse

Author (Year)	Indication	Number of Patients	Follow-Up	Outcome
Alnaif and Drutz (2000)[21]	Pessary use and changes in vaginal flora	220	0.5–8 years	Increased odds of bacterial vaginosis (odds ratio [OR] 4.37)
Robert and Mainprize (2002)[22]	Acceptance to pessary for treatment of stress urinary incontinence	38	12 months	16% continuation
Lazarou et al. (2004)[1]	Relief of urinary retention with pessary use and predicting resolution of retention after reconstructive surgery in women with anterior vaginal prolapse	24	3 months postoperatively	Positive predictive value of 94% and negative predictive value of 67%
Donnelly et al. (2004)[23]	Stress and mixed urinary incontinence	119	6 months	89% successful fitting, 52% continued use
Fernando et al. (2006)[24]	Effects of pessary on symptoms associated with prolapse	203	4 months	75% successful fitting, 40% improved voiding, 28% improved bowel evacuation, 26% of sexually active patients with improved frequency and 11% with improved satisfaction
Cundiff et al. (2007)[25]	Patient satisfaction between the two most common pessaries: Gellhorn and ring with support	134	3 months	Improvement in relieving symptoms with both pessaries, no significant difference between the two pessaries
Richter et al. (2010)[8]	Compare the effectiveness of a continence pessary to behavioral therapy to combined pessary and behavioral therapy for treatment of stress incontinence	446	3, 6, and 12 months	At 3 months, satisfaction of treatment was 63% in pessary, 75% in behavioral, and 79% in combined group; treatment success declined in all groups at 12 months; overall treatment satisfaction remained >50% in all three groups at 12 months
Abdool et al. (2011)[26]	Compare the effectiveness of pessary and surgery in women with symptomatic prolapse	554	1 year	Improvement in prolapse, urinary, bowel, and sexual function in both groups without significant difference
Ramsay et al. (2016)[27]	Outcomes of pessary use in older women	304		Erosion rate of 18.3% in long-term users, age ≥75 years were more likely to have erosions
Coolen et al. (2018)[28]	Compare the functional outcomes after pessary versus surgery for treatment of prolapse	113	12 months	In pessary group, expulsion 14%, discharge 20%, vaginal pain 14%, incontinence 9%, erosion 4%, 28% surgical intervention

TABLE 6.2

Impact of Pessary Use on Quality of Life (QOL)

Author	QOL Impact	Number of Patients	Follow-Up	Outcome
Patel et al. (2010)[29]	Prolapse symptoms, QOL, and body image	75	3 months	Significant reduction of bothersome symptoms, improvement of QOL and body image
Brazell et al. (2014)[30]	Change in bowel symptoms	104	12 months	Significant improvements in both bowel-related symptoms and bowel-related QOL
Lone et al. (2015)[31]	Outcomes of pessaries and surgery in women with symptomatic pelvic organ prolapse (POP)	287	1 year	Nonbothersome symptom of vaginal soreness in the pessary group and the symptom of a tight vagina in the surgery group; overall, statistically significant difference in improvement in vaginal, sex, QOL, and urinary symptom scores in both groups and no difference between the two groups
Meriwether et al. (2015)[13]	Sexual function	127	3 months	No difference in sexual function before and after the pessary placement; significant improvement in self-consciousness; majority of sexually active women removed their pessary for sex
Cheung et al. (2016)[10]	Pelvic floor symptoms, QOL, and complications with or without vaginal pessaries	276	12 months	Prolapse symptoms and quality of life were improved in women using a vaginal pessary
Ai et al. (2018)[9]	Effect of generalized anxiety disorders (GADs) on the success of pessary treatment for pelvic organ prolapse	21	3 months	Both groups of women with or without GADs showed significant improvement in QOL scores after 3 months of pessary treatment; GADs had no influence on the success of pessary treatment for POP
Ai et al. (2018)[9]	Depressive symptoms on successful pessary treatment	102	3 months	Both the QOL and depressive symptom scores were significantly improved after 3 months of successful pessary use

complications, such as severe erosions or fistula formation, are uncommon, and 91% of these complications are related to neglected pessaries.[15]

In order to prevent these complications, it is necessary for patients follow-up with their provider regularly. Although there are no clear guidelines regarding pessary care, some experts recommend follow-up 1–3 days after initial placement, then at 4–6 weeks depending on the patient's ability to manage the pessary, and every 6–12 months after that.[16] Despite these recommendations by many practitioners, there has not been an association demonstrated between the frequency of pessary changes and complications.[11] Women can choose to provide self-care, removing their pessary periodically or before intercourse. These women are advised to remove the pessary and clean it with soap and water, and they should be followed at regular intervals.[17] Alternatively, women may choose to have their pessary maintenance managed by their health care provider. Provider maintenance typically occurs every 3 months consisting of a pelvic exam to assess for erosions, irritation, and possible significant complications. Compared to those fitted with a support pessary, provider maintenance is more common in those fitted with a space-occupying pessary. Therefore, in order to prevent and detect complications, patients desiring pessary use must be able to adhere to the recommended follow-up.

Changes in the vaginal microenvironment from pessary use have also been described. Bacterial vaginosis is more common in pessary users (32%) compared to nonusers (10%).[15] A secondary analysis of a multicenter randomized trial of hydroxyquinoline gel in women presenting for pessary fitting showed that the frequency of pessary changes also affects this microenvironment. This analysis found that women who removed their pessary less than weekly were more likely to have anaerobic predominance at 3 months. In addition, a predominance of lactobacillus was higher in those who removed their pessary daily (41% daily, 24% weekly, 9% longer, $P = .03$). However, vaginal symptoms and pessary satisfaction did not differ among these groups.[18]

Predictors for Unsuccessful Fitting and Reasons for Discontinuation

The predictors for unsuccessful fitting and reasons for discontinuation can be found in Table 6.3. Fitting is successful in 62% of patients. However, significant barriers to successful fitting included short vaginal length (≤ 6 cm) and a wide introitus (>4 fingerbreadths).[19] Other predictors of unsuccessful fitting include a history of prior surgery for prolapse or hysterectomy.[20]

Most patients who are successfully fitted for a pessary continue with its use. However, some factors increase the likelihood for discontinuation, such as worsening or occult stress urinary incontinence, increased discharge,

TABLE 6.3

Reasons for Discontinuation and/or Failure to Retain

Author	Number of Patients	Follow-Up	Outcome	Reason for Discontinuation
Clemons et al. (2004)[32]	100	1 week, 2 months	73% with successful 2-week pessary fitting trial and majority with resolution of prolapse-related symptoms; ring pessaries more with stage II and III prolapse, Gellhorn pessaries with stage IV prolapse	Dissatisfaction associated with occult stress incontinence; unsuccessful fitting: short vaginal length and wide introitus were risk factors for failure
Mutone et al. (2005)[33]	407	3 weeks	41% successfully fitted and continued use at 3 weeks	Hysterectomy and known surgery for prolapse a risk factor for unsuccessful fitting; there was no association between the stage of prolapse and pessary trial outcome
Nguyen et al. (2005)[36]	130	28–69 months	63% successfully fitted; of the successfully fitted patients, 50% discontinued by 24 months	Unsuccessful fitting: previous prolapse repair, presence of stress urinary incontinence
Bai et al. (2005)[15]	104	6 months	80.9% continuation rate; 70.2% patients satisfied or very satisfied	Erosion, bleeding, discharge, discomfort, and slipping
Maito et al. (2006)[20]		6 months	86% successfully fitted; 89% continued use at 6 months	Severe posterior prolapse
Fernando et al. (2006)[24]	203	4 months	75% retention	Failure to retain: increased parity, prior hysterectomy
Komesu et al. (2008)[35]	64	2, 6, and 12 months	56% continued use	
Coolen et al. (2018)[28] (pessary versus surgery)	113	12 months	60% at 12 months	Expulsion, incontinence, vaginal pain, vaginal discharge, no improvement in symptoms

discomfort, and lack of improvement in symptoms. Significant posterior prolapse has also been shown to result in discontinuation.[20]

Conclusion

Pessaries can serve as a safe, long-term, conservative option for management of pelvic organ prolapse and stress urinary incontinence in a selected group of patients. Although the continuation of and satisfaction with a pessary depend on many individual patient factors, a pessary should be offered as management to all patients with prolapse and stress urinary incontinence symptoms regardless of their initial management desires. It must be offered even to those with no contraindication to surgery; however, they must understand that a pessary is not a permanent or definitive solution to their problem but instead requires a long-term management plan. The pessary has the ability to not only improve symptoms but also to avoid the risks associated with surgery. In addition, it can provide diagnostic and predictive information for patients contemplating surgery. The sum of all the benefits of pessary use makes this device a useful option in many patients.

REFERENCES

1. Lazarou G, Scotti RJ, Mikhail MS, Zhou HS, Powers K. Pessary reduction and postoperative cure of retention in women with anterior vaginal wall prolapse. *Int Urogynecol J.* 2004;15(3):175–178.
2. Ding J, Chen C, Song XC, Zhang L, Deng M, Zhu L. Changes in prolapse and urinary symptoms after successful fitting of a ring pessary with support in women with advanced pelvic organ prolapse: A prospective study. *Urology.* 2016;87:70–75.
3. Sung VW, Wohlrab KJ, Madsen A, Raker C. Patient-reported goal attainment and comprehensive functioning outcomes after surgery compared to pessary for pelvic organ prolapse. *Am J Obstet Gynecol.* 2016;215(5):659.e1–659.e7.
4. Clemons JL, Aguilar VC, Tillinghast TA, Jackson ND, Myers DL. Patient satisfaction and changes in prolapse and urinary symptoms in women who were fitted successfully with a pessary for pelvic organ prolapse. *Am J Obstet Gynecol.* 2004;190(4):1025–1029.
5. Wood LN, Anger JT. Urinary incontinence in women. *BMJ.* 2014;349:g4531.
6. Karan A, Aksac B, Attar E et al. Hypermobility syndrome in 105 women with pure urinary stress incontinence and in 105 controls. *Arch Gynecol Obstet.* 2004;269(2):89–90.
7. Farrell SA, Singh B, Aldakhil L. Continence pessaries in the management of urinary incontinence in women. *J Obstet Gynecol Can.* 2004;26(2):113–117.
8. Richter HE, Burgio KL, Brubaker L et al. Continence pessary compared with behavioral therapy or combined therapy for stress incontinence: A randomized controlled trial. *Obstet Gynecol.* 2010;115(3):609–617.
9. Ai FF, Zhu L, Mao M, Zhang Y, Kang J. Depressive symptoms affect outcomes of pessary use in postmenopausal women with uterine prolapse. *Climacteric.* 2018;21(2):184-188.

10. Cheung RY, Lee JH, Lee LL, Chung TK, Chan SS. Vaginal pessary in women with symptomatic pelvic organ prolapse: A randomized controlled trial. *Obstet Gynecol.* 2016;128(1):73–80.
11. Tenfelde S, Tell D, Thomas TN, Kenton K. Quality of life in women who use pessaries for longer than 12 months. *Female Pelvic Med Reconstr Surg.* 2015;21(3):146–149.
12. Brincat C, Kenton K, Pat Fitzgerald M, Brubaker L. Sexual activity predicts continued pessary use. *Am J Obstet Gynecol.* 2004;191(1):198–200.
13. Meriwether KV, Komesu YM, Craig E, Qualls C, Davis H, Rogers RG. Sexual function and pessary management among women using a pessary for pelvic floor disorders. *J Sex Med.* 2015;12(12):2339–2349.
14. Hason LM, Schulz JA, Flood CG et al. Vaginal pessaries in managing women with pelvic organ prolapse and urinary incontinence: Patient characteristics and factors contributing to success. *Int Urogynecol J.* 2006;17(2):155–159.
15. Bai SW, Yoon BS, Kwon JY, Shin JS, Kim SK, Park KH. Survey of the characteristics and satisfaction degree of the patients using a pessary. *Int Urogynecol J Pelvic Floor Dysfunct.* 2005;16(3):182–186.
16. Karam M, Walters M (Eds.). Stress urinary incontinence and pelvic organ prolapse: Nonsurgical management. In: *Urogynecology and Reconstructive Pelvic Surgery*, 4th edition, 2014: pp. 250–251. Philadelphia: Elsevier.
17. Robert M, Schulz JA, Harvey MA. Technical update on pessary use. *J Obstet. Gynaecol Canada.* 2013;35(7):664–674.
18. Fregosi NJ, Hobson DTG, Kinman CL, Gaskins JT, Stewart JR, Meriwether KV. Changes in the vaginal microenvironment as related to frequency of pessary removal. *Female Pelvic Med Reconstr Surg.* 2018;24(2):166–171.
19. Manchana T. Ring pessary for pelvic organ prolapse. *Arch Gynecol Obstet.* 2011;284(2):391–395.
20. Maito JM, Quam ZA, Craig E, Danner KA, Rogers RG. Predictors of successful pessary fitting and continued use in a nurse-midwifery pessary clinic. *J Midwifery Women's Health.* 2006;51(2):78–84.
21. Alnaif B, Drutz HP. Bacterial vaginosis increases in pessary users. *Int Urogynecol J Pelvic Floor Dysfunct.* 2000;11(4):219–222.
22. Robert M, Mainprize TC. Long-term assessment of the incontinence ring pessary for the treatment of stress incontinence. *Int Urogynecol J.* 2002;13(5):236–239.
23. Donnelly MJ, Powell-Morgan S, Olsen AL, Nygaard IE. Vaginal pessaries for the management of stress and mixed urinary incontinence. *Int Urogencol J Pelvic Floor Dysfunct.* 2004;15(5):302–307.
24. Fernando RJ, Thakar R, Sultan AH, Shah SM, Jones PW. Effect of vaginal pessaries on symptoms associated with pelvic organ prolapse. *Obstet Gynecol.* 2006;108(1):93–99.
25. Cundiff GW, Amundsen CL, Bent AE et al. The PESSRI study: Symptom relief outcomes of a randomized crossover trial of the ring and Gellhorn pessaries. *AJOG.* 2007;196(4):405.e1–405.e8.
26. Abdool Z, Thakar R, Sultan AH, Oliver RS. Prospective evaluation of outcome of vaginal pessaries versus surgery in women with symptomatic pelvic organ prolapse. *Int Urogynecol J.* 2011;22(3):273–278.
27. Ramsay S, Tu LM, Tannenbaum C. Natural history of pessary use in women aged 65–74 versus 75 years and older with pelvic organ prolapse: A 12-year study. *Int Urogynecol J.* 2016;27(8):1201–1207.

28. Coolen, AWM, Troost S, Mol BWJ, Roovers JPWR, Bongers MY. Primary treatment of pelvic organ prolapse: Pessary use versus prolapse surgery. *Int Urogynecol J.* 2018;29(1):99–107.

29. Patel M, Mellen C, O'Sullivan DM, LaSala CA. Impact of pessary use on prolapse symptoms, quality of life, and body image. *Am J Obstet Gynecol.* 2010;202(5):499.e1–499.e4.

30. Brazell HD, Patel M, O'Sullivan DM, Mellen C, LaSala CA. The impact of pessary use on bowel symptoms: One-year outcomes. *Female Pelvic Med Reconstr Surg.* 2014;20(2):95–98.

31. Lone F, Thakar R, Sultan AH. One-year prospective comparison of vaginal pessaries and surgery for pelvic organ prolapse using the validated ICIQ-vS and ICIQ-UI (SF) questionnaires. *Int Urogynecol J.* 2015;26(9):1305–1312.

32. Clemons JL, Aguilar VC, Tillinghast TA, Jackson ND, Myers DL. Risk factors associated with an unsuccessful pessary fitting trial in women with pelvic organ prolapse. *Am J Obstet Gynecol.* 2004;190(2):345–350.

33. Mutone MF, Terry C, Hale DS, Benson JT. Factors which influence the short-term success of pessary management of pelvic organ prolapse. *Am J Obstet Gynecol.* 2005;193(1):89–94.

34. Nguyen JN, Jones CR. Pessary treatment of pelvic relaxation: Factors affecting successful fitting and continued use. *J Wound Ostomy Continence Nurs.* 2005;32(4):255–261.

35. Komesu YM, Rogers RG, Rode MA, Craig EC, Schrader RM, Gallegos KA, Villareal B. Patient-selected goal attainment for pessary wearers: What is the clinical relevance? *Am J Obstet Gynecol.* 2008;198(5):577–585.

7

Current Clinical Studies in Vaginal Pessaries

Kelly Jirschele

CONTENTS

Pessary Uses for Pelvic Organ Prolapse

As this text thoroughly describes, pessary management has been an option to address symptoms of pelvic organ prolapse (POP) for years. Pessaries offer a conservative, low-morbidity management option for controlling prolapse symptoms. They provide low complication rates, while follow-up management strategies minimize complications.

Most current studies in pessary use for POP focus on patterns of use and predictors of discontinuation.[1,2] Alperin et al. using diagnostic and procedural codes reviewed a random national sample of Medicare and Medicaid service beneficiaries to identify women with POP that were treated with a pessary. They found that more than 11% of women in the sample with POP were treated with a pessary. By the end of the first year, 12% of these women had surgery for POP, and by the end of their study at 9 years, 24% had surgery. As this was a study using codes, not actual charts, there is no further explanation of why these women ultimately chose surgery to manage their POP.

Dengler et al. reviewed charts of all women undergoing pessary fitting at one institution. They defined defecatory dysfunction as constipation, straining, splinting, or incomplete evacuation. In these patients, the overall pessary discontinuation rate was 77% and statistical analysis using a logistic regression model identified incomplete defecation as the most significant factor associated with pessary discontinuation. They concluded that perhaps better understanding of pessary discontinuation factors could help direct treatment options.

Pessary use has been shown to significantly improve pelvic floor symptoms as measured by the Prolapse and Urinary Scales of the Pelvic Floor Distress Inventory.[3] Despite the potential for low-risk symptom improvement with using a pessary, discontinuation is common. Pessaries can cause an odorous discharge, which may be bothersome to patients. Defecatory dysfunction is also strongly associated with discontinuation.[2] Mao et al. suggest that while pessary use is safe and effective, defecatory symptoms often persist, and this may lead to discontinuation.[2,4]

Mao et al. prospectively followed successfully patients fitted with a ring pessary with support. They used validated tools to follow patients' symptoms and quality of life. While there were improvements in prolapse and urinary incontinence symptoms, there was no significant improvement in defecatory symptoms.

In a study from 2009, Sarma et al. found during follow-up that the majority of women elected to stop using a pessary. Depending on how one defines a complication (bleeding, extrusion, vaginal discharge, pain, and constipation), 56% of woman studied had at least one complication. Some would argue that these are not all true complications, but pessary continuation in this study was only 14%.[5]

Jones and Harmanli investigated how improvements in pessary design may lead to improved long-term use.[6] They suggested that given the aging population, pessary use may be gaining interest as a conservative option to manage women's pelvic floor disorders. One of the novel ideas in pessary design was a new device that helps improve pelvic floor strength with its use. Another new concept was the use of a pessary that includes a handle at the pessary base.[6] Unfortunately, other than these innovations, not much has currently changed with pessary styles, and while these ideas are promising, to date, none have made a dramatic change in pessary use practice in the United States.

There is a disposable product under investigation in the United States. The ProVate device is a single-use ring pessary device deployed with a vaginal applicator (Figure 7.1). The device has a narrow insertion dimension and expands laterally in the vagina. Like a tampon, it has a string for easy removal and disposal. It offers a conservative approach providing temporary relief of POP symptoms while improving long-term pessary use.

Other than the mainstream use of pessaries, some are being used for novel treatments. An interesting case report discusses the use of the Gellhorn pessary to support prolapse in a cervical cancer patient with procidentia to help facilitate chemotherapy and radiation.[7] More recently, there has been a discussion of customizing the manufacturing of pessaries with three-dimensional printing. Barsky et al. offered this twenty-first century concept as an option for patients with anatomical variation making traditional pessary fitting challenging.[8]

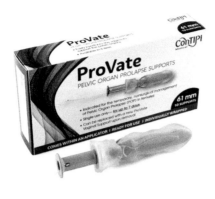

FIGURE 7.1 The ProVate pessary is shown here with vaginal applicator. This disposable, single-use pessary has a string attached as shown for ease of removal. (Courtesy of Dr. Elan Ziv.)

Pessary Uses for Stress Urinary Incontinence

Vaginal pessary use for stress urinary incontinence (SUI) is effective when fitted appropriately and managed well. Al-Shaikh et al. noted that vaginal pessaries are an effective SUI management option and feel they should be considered a first-line treatment for symptomatic patients.[9] Vaginal pessaries for urinary incontinence support the urethra and work to control leakage with an increase in intra-abdominal pressure. There are commercially available disposable products that also provide support and work to control leakage with activity using the same concept. These products are marketed as a relatively new, over-the-counter option for SUI management. These products work to support the urethra like pessaries designed for incontinence. These are made of soft, flexible silicone enclosed in a nonabsorbent covering and easily inserted into the vagina with a tampon-like applicator. Data provided by the manufacturer suggest most patients report significant leak reduction using these vaginal inserts.[10] Uresta incontinence pessary (Figure 7.2) (Halifax, Nova Scotia, Canada) is a bladder support product marketed to help control leakage with activity. It has a bell-shaped design with a handle for ease of use and a tapered tip to allow for vaginal introduction. The bell shape allows for support at the urethra. This product can be reused for up to 1 year before the recommended replacement.[11]

Women using a pessary may feel less self-conscious, contributing to improved sexual function. This finding is based on questionnaire data and the work aimed to describe sexual function among pessary users. These women completed the Pelvic Organ Prolapse–Urinary Incontinence Sexual Function Questionnaire,

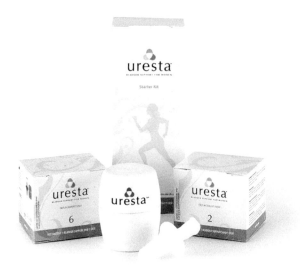

FIGURE 7.2   The Uresta incontinence pessary, to attempt to reduce urinary leakage.

International Urogynecological Association Revised (PISQ-IR), a validated measure that evaluates the impact of pelvic floor disorders on sexual function, a modified female body image scale (mBIS), and questions regarding pessary management surrounding sexual activity. Scores improved in the questions related to self-consciousness. Pessary satisfaction was associated with improved sexual function scores in multiple domains and improved mBIS scores.[12]

In a prospective observational study, total vaginal length ≥7.5 cm and a higher baseline Pelvic Organ Prolapse Distress Inventory 6 score were independent factors associated with long-term pessary use after successful fitting in women with symptomatic POP. They aimed to evaluate the continuation rate and identify the factors related to long-term pessary use. The median follow-up time on these 277 women successfully fit with pessary was 26 months. At the study endpoint, 76.5% of patients continued to use pessaries.[13]

Pessary Use for Preterm Birth

The majority of data in the literature focusing on current clinical studies with pessaries are related to cervical pessaries and their use in the prevention of preterm delivery. New studies are published nearly every month. Obstetricians are excited about the potential for a low-morbidity option to help manage the challenging predicament of preterm birth, especially related to cervical incompetence. Unfortunately, the data are mixed, and no clear guidelines or recommendations exist for use. Cervical pessaries are used in cases of cervical insufficiency and are placed to aid in keeping the cervix closed.